G. Timothy Johnson, M.D.

DOCTOR!

What You Should Know about Health Care *Before* You Call a Physician

McGraw-Hill Book Company

NEW YORK   ST. LOUIS   SAN FRANCISCO   DÜSSELDORF

LONDON   MEXICO   SYDNEY   TORONTO

Designed by Lynn Braswell.

123456789BPBP798765

Library of Congress Cataloging in Publication Data

Johnson, G   Timothy.
    Doctor!
    1. Physician and patient. 2. Medical care.
3. Medicine, Popular. I. Title. [DNLM: 1. Medicine
—Popular works.   WB120 J67d]
R727.3.J64   610   74-31459
ISBN 0-07-032664-9
ISBN 0-07-032663-0 pbk.

Contents

[If you need to use this book in an emergency, turn to the **INDEX** (page 403). Treatments for such emergency situations as **Burns, Collapse, Poisoning,** etc., are listed alphabetically, with appropriate page references, in bold, prominent type.]

Introduction   1

PART I   *A Quick Guide to the Health Care*
             Market   5

Choosing a Hospital   7
Evaluating Doctors   15
The Scorecard   21
Primary Care   39
Changing Practice Patterns   43
Choosing a Doctor   47
The Question of Surgery   51
Doctors and Money   59
When to See a Doctor   67
How a Doctor Thinks   73

v

A618253

PART II   *Common Medical Problems*   79

   1. *Emergencies*   85
   2. *Heart Disease*   115
   3. *Lung Disease*   141
   4. *Cancer*   151
   5. *Gastrointestinal Disease*   159
   6. *Infectious Disease*   187
   7. *Nutrition*   195
   8. *Women's Health Problems*   211
   A Dictionary of Other Health Problems   241

PART III   *Looking Ahead at American Health
                    Care*   387

Bibliography   399

Index   403

Introduction

This book has two purposes: (1) to summarize significant health information, and (2) to provide a guide to health care where choices may be important.

The book grows out of my experience in dealing with the concerns of medical consumers—meaning anyone who has ever sought medical care—both as a practicing emergency room physician and as a practicing "television doctor." The latter activity has exposed me to a wide range of concerns and has sharpened my understanding of the medical information needs of the so-called "average person." The book also reflects my growing conviction that one of the best ways to change health care is to better inform the potential patient. An informed patient will get better medical care—and that will effect change.

As the title indicates, this book is a *guide, not* another home medical encyclopedia or first aid manual. It deliberately avoids comprehensive descriptions of all health problems. Instead, this is an attempt to gather together from the enormous mountain of health information those items which *everyone* should know about. I have been guided by the following questions in my selection: What new information is really worth knowing? What old information is still important and what should be discarded? What are the facts about the important controversies in medicine—treatment for breast cancer, vitamins, the role of coronary bypass surgery, etc.? What "preventive medicine" should everyone practice? What general principles and specific pitfalls of health care choices should everybody know about?

In other words, this book is highly selective, and the following kinds of information are *not* to be found:

1. Complete discussions of any specific disease. Although some health problems are discussed in considerable detail, persons with a very specific medical problem will need more information. (A brief bibliography of good sources of lay health information appears at the end of the book.)

2. Specifics about costs, insurance programs, federal legislation, etc. Such details are changing so fast that anything now printed will soon be out of date. I do, however, highlight general principles and specific dangers in choosing health care.

3. Treatment of uncommon or esoteric health problems. My selection is based in part on the degree of general interest. Unusual topics must be sought elsewhere.

4. Details concerning childhood health development. This book is primarily about adult health problems, though several common childhood problems are included.

5. Discussions on diseases which are common and significant but for which no new information of great significance is available—e.g., multiple sclerosis.

Also, it should be made clear that this book is written for those in our society who are fortunate enough to be able to choose health care. I am painfully aware that many in our society are so limited by poverty, geography, ignorance, time, and sex (women, in general, have more difficulty in dealing with the medical establishment) that the possibility of "choosing medical care" is largely, for them, a myth. I recognize that this book—which assumes the possibility of choices—will be of little direct help for such people. I can only hope that, to the degree that this book contributes to changes in health care for those who can choose, such care will also be changed for those who must accept whatever is offered.

The book is divided into three sections. Part I deals with some basic issues in choosing medical care, including the selection of a doctor. Part II discusses specific medical problems. Part III—"Looking Ahead"—discusses issues that affect health care but are at least once removed from you and me as individual consumers. You should read this section first to discover some of my biases.

I wrote the book to be read in its entirety. It may be used as a reference or in a "pick and choose" manner, but I hope that most readers will take the time to read it through. I would like to think they will be reasonably well-informed medical consumers as a result. I am completely responsible for the content and selection in this book. I have asked specialist friends to check appropriate parts for accuracy, but the final result is my responsibility.

Finally, a reminder that your good health is largely up to you—and not the "health care industry" or your doctor.

Many major causes of illness and disability in this country —accidents, drinking, smoking, overeating—are under your control. As a medical consumer, let alone the one most interested in your own health, you should strive to remember that good health literally does begin at home.

G. Timothy Johnson, M.D.

P.S. Throughout the book I use masculine pronouns. This is done out of habit and in the interest of efficiency. I wish here to acknowledge clearly the growing role of women physicians and to express my own opinion that women have indeed been the object of real (though usually unintentional) discrimination by the male establishment of medicine.

A Quick Guide to the Health Care Market

As they say at the ballpark, you can't tell the players without a scorecard. This section is designed to provide you with a brief scorecard for the world of medical care. There is a certain logic to the order of topics, but they can also be read independently according to your need for specific information. The final section, "How a Doctor Thinks," provides an insider's insight into the thinking and feeling of the typical doctor as he encounters a patient.

Choosing a Hospital

It might seem strange to start a scorecard with buildings instead of people. But, in modern society, hospitals have become the focal point for health personnel—including doctors. And one of the best ways to choose doctors is first to choose a good hospital and then choose the appropriate doctor on its staff. Selecting a "good" hospital is not that easy. Hospitals are complex institutions and are usually a mixed bag of good and bad. The nursing may be excellent but the food terrible. The X-ray department may be superb but the laboratory only adequate. And, for the average medical consumer without authoritative inside information, a total evaluation of any given hospital is almost impossible.

However, choosing a hospital for the specific purpose of selecting a doctor on its staff is more manageable. The concern now becomes the general medical reputation of a hospital in terms of the quality of doctors on its staff. There are some general guidelines which may be useful.

Accreditation by the JCAH (Joint Commission on Accreditation of Hospitals)

This is a useful check only in avoiding (like the plague) hospitals that do not have such accreditation. Such accreditation provides that minimal standards of care—as determined by an investigating team, usually every two years—are being met. It does *not* guarantee quality physician care. It *does* protect against overcrowding, unsanitary conditions, etc.

More recently, the Joint Commission (so-called because it represents a cooperative venture of several important health groups) has been moving into more meaningful areas of physician evaluation, such as actual analysis of how physicians perform in treating certain diseases. That kind of analysis is not yet reflected in the awarding of accreditation. You can find out if a given hospital has JCAH accreditation by asking the hospital administrator or writing to the JCAH at: 875 N. Michigan Ave., Chicago, Ill. 60611.

Teaching Hospitals

One of the quickest ways to be reasonably assured of a source of quality physicians is to turn to a so-called "teaching hospital." Ideally, all hospitals should be halls of learning, where doctors and other members of the health care team are always improving. But this phrase is usually used in a more technical sense to describe hospitals that have a formal affiliation with a medical school. Sometimes that affiliation is obvious by name or location. Quite often, however, such a linkage may not be so obvious, and you need to ask the question: Is this hospital affiliated with a medical school and, if so, how? The degree of affiliation can vary considerably, from the hospital totally under the control of a medical school to a community hospital through which some medical students rotate for part of their educational experience. Generally, any small community hospital which trumpets itself as a teaching hospital is overstating its case.

Another sign of a teaching hospital is the presence of interns (physicians in their first year after medical school) and residents (physicians in specialty training). Interns and residents are often referred to collectively as "house staff." Their presence means, among other things, that physicians on staff at that hospital are more likely to be "kept on their toes" and stimulated by the presence of learning and inquiring minds.

Why all this fuss about "teaching hospitals"? Because, generally speaking, teaching hospitals have higher standards both in accepting physicians on staff and in setting limitations on what they may do. Some important qualifications should be stated immediately, however. Like any other hospital, even a teaching hospital tends to keep physicians on staff beyond quality limits on age, skills, or knowledge. And often admission to staff status is as much a matter of politics as ability; some teaching hospitals have what amounts to a closed shop, and not being appointed to such a staff does not mean that ability was the issue. Also, some teaching hospitals have developed an arrogant attitude which falsely suggests that only their doctors and their methods are acceptable.

Further, teaching hospitals may have real disadvantages in providing the niceties of patient care, especially if they are large and impersonal. But I am now talking only about physician selection, and the initial statement still stands. One of the quickest ways to reasonably assure a source of quality physicians is to turn to a "teaching hospital." This statement does *not* mean that quality physicians cannot be found elsewhere. It just means this is one way of zeroing in quickly.

Nonprofit Community vs. Proprietary Hospital

Another quick way to avoid physicians of lesser ability is to avoid proprietary hospitals—privately owned, for-profit hospitals. This is an obvious generalization with many exceptions, but common sense dictates that profit considerations may not always be synonymous with concerns for quality care.

The vast majority of hospitals in this country, including most teaching hospitals, fall into the category of "nonprofit, community." This simply means that the alleged purpose of the hospital is other than to make a profit for stockholders or owners. Clearly such a designation says nothing about the quality of physicians.

A third category of hospitals should be mentioned, namely, "public" hospitals operated by municipal, state, or federal government. Hospitals in this category vary widely in quality (as is true of the other two categories mentioned), but they generally offer competent medical services in a setting devoid of "niceties." Some large municipal or county hospitals perform a tremendous service to inner-city residents but often do so in a manner that antagonizes recipients of care. Many large teaching hospitals under the control of medical schools are financed and operated by government.

The fact of the matter is that most people choose a hospital on the basis of geographical convenience; in some rural areas, there is no such choice. But in urban areas with available transportation, it pays to start one's search for a doctor with a search for a "good" hospital. Which brings us back to where we started in this section.

Signposts of a "Good" Hospital

Limiting yourself to the question of the quality of physicians on its staff, you can, in evaluating a hospital, specifically explore the following questions:

1. What is the percentage of board-certified physicians on the staff? (We'll be exploring the meaning of "board certification" in the next section.)

2. What departments (medicine, surgery, etc.) have "fulltime chiefs"? A "fulltime chief" refers to a physician who spends all of his professional time working for and in the hospital—versus also maintaining a private practice outside the hospital. Such an arrangement is no guarantee of quality, but a department with a fulltime chief is more likely to have an on-going quality control over what takes place on that service.

3. What kind of education programs are provided for the staff? Is attendance at such programs required to maintain staff privileges? Do the doctors take an active role in the continuing education of nurses and other health personnel in the hospital?

4. What kind of review exists for the work of physicians on the staff? Are tissues removed at surgery reviewed for the necessity of surgery and are surgeons corrected? Does the medical service check on the care of heart attack victims? Is there any provision for supervision of physicians who are not board certified? Does the hospital have ways of identifying the physician who has become incompetent?

In other words, you should ask questions that probe the "medical environment" (versus the physical plant) of the hospital. You should ask questions that attempt to answer this question: Does the medical staff have an active and creative concern to improve the level of its practice, or is it content to maintain the status quo?

We now come to the biggest question of all. Whom do you ask? How do you get honest answers to these and similar questions? Some of the information is a matter of facts and can be obtained by direct inquiry of the hospital's administrative office. (You can make a list of your questions and either write or call; some hospitals have printed information available concerning the structure and activity of their medical staff.) But, even after obtaining "official" information, it would be highly useful to get some "inside" information concerning doctors and hospitals in your area.

Obtaining Inside Information

It is important to underscore that what I mean by "inside" information is *not* some hidden cache of facts which hospitals and/or doctors are attempting to keep from the public. (Like all humans and human institutions, doctors and hospitals will generally try to put their best foot forward, and in so doing they may be misleading.) Rather, I am talking about the kind of "information"—more properly described as "gossip"—that exists on the inside of any institution. There are real dangers in accepting "gossip" as "gospel." But there are also real rewards in taking the time to sift through such gossip for pearls of information that may be useful.

What you should look for are people who work in a hospital and have an opportunity to observe the work of doctors. If you have a close friend or relative who is a doctor, that may be a useful source of information about other doctors. But most doctors are not in a position to observe the work and manner of most other physicians. The exception to this is a doctor who works fulltime in the hospital (see the later section on hospital-based physicians, pp. 35–37); such a doctor—radiologist, pathologist, anesthesiologist, etc.—may be an excellent source of opinion *if* your relationship with that doctor is such that you can expect a candid opinion.

Most people, however, do not have access to such physicians. But there are many other hospital personnel who do have the opportunity to assess medical care in a hospital. I am going to list some of them with the suggestion that, if you look in your neighborhood or circle of acquaintances, you are very likely to find one of the following excellent sources of information:

1. Nurses: Probably the best source of information, since they work most closely with doctors.

2. Operating-room technicians: An excellent source of information on various surgeons.

3. X-ray and laboratory technicians: Less direct contact with doctors, but they hear about what goes on in a hospital.

4. Respiratory technicians (inhalation therapists): Considerable opportunity to observe what goes on inside hospitals.

5. Physical therapists: Opportunity for observation similar to inhalation therapists.

6. Etc., etc.: In large hospitals, there are many other employees who have opportunity to become acquainted

with the quality of the medical staff—in general and in particular. I suggest that if you look and ask, you are likely to find a reliable inside source from among the above—on your street, in your church, a member of your club, etc. You will obviously have to evaluate the source of your information. But, if the person has worked in a given hospital for a reasonable length of time and if that person is willing to share choices that he makes for himself, such information could be very useful. Obviously the best time to make such an investigation is *before* an illness strikes . . . while there is time.

Evaluating Doctors

Training and Boards

You should understand that all states will license a physician to practice (if he can pass certain requirements) after four years of medical school plus one year of internship; a few states do not even require the internship to become eligible for licensing. Once licensed, a physician can call himself anything he wants. For example, even if a physician has no training beyond internship, he can call himself a cardiologist, or a psychiatrist—or even a surgeon. (The title "physician and surgeon" is a traditional designation for the general practitioner and is still found on many signs and diplomas.) Fortunately, there are some practical limitations on this practice of designation without training. The most important limitation is that of a good hospital which determines what each physician may do within its walls. But a physician who confines his practice to his office has no similar review, and only under the most dreadful of circumstances will he be investigated by the state licensing authority. In other words, the holding of "a license to practice medicine" tells you nothing about a given physician's training, other than the fact that he holds an M.D. degree for which he qualified after four years of medical school.

Another way to check on competency is to see if the physician is "Board certified" in the specialty he claims. Each specialty has a "board" (meaning regulatory staff) which supervises training and certifies competency. A physician who passes the examination of a given specialty is known as a diplomate of that board and is said to be board certified. Actual certification *may* not be critical. Older specialists often trained under a kind of preceptorship system and may not have official certification. Others may have completed a formal training program (residency) and are said to be "board eligible" (eligible to "take their boards" or certifying exams) but either have chosen not to take the exams or failed the exams and decided not to try again. To fail specialty exams is not *always* as bad as it sounds; some specialties have a built-in failure percentage for each exam, and some exams have been notorious for subjectivity on the part of the examiners. I know of well-trained specialists who for one legitimate reason or another are not actually certified. But these are exceptions; it is "better to have passed than not to have passed."

Another check on quality is membership in a "college" —the honorary membership group of a given specialty. Such membership is acquired only after certain requirements have been met. The initials after a doctor's name usually indicate such membership—such as FACS, for "Fellow in the American College of Surgeons." Don't accept strange initials after a name until you check to see what they mean.

Information concerning training can be obtained from several sources. If you are new in town and searching for a physician, I would not hesitate to question the office nurse or secretary regarding credentials. However, it may be less embarrassing to make such inquiries of the local or state medical society; if they do not have the information readily at hand, you may ask them to inquire for you and then call again. The key questions to ask:

1. Where and when did the physician do his post–medical school training—internship and residency?

2. Is he board certified or board eligible? (*The Directory of Medical Specialists* provides a listing of diplomates of the twenty-two specialties in this country. The latest edition—the sixteenth—can be found in many public libraries.)

3. Is the physician a member of the appropriate specialty "college"?

4. What hospitals is he affiliated with?

5. What teaching appointments—if any—does he have?

6. What papers—if any—has he published?

The answers to these questions may or may not be important. Some publishing and teaching accomplishments mean little; others point to real achievement. And positive answers to all the above do not guarantee competency. But they are factors to consider when choosing a physician.

Continuing Education

I now come to one of the most difficult areas to evaluate —namely, how to tell if a given physician has "kept up." As with any kind of evaluation, one is dealing with that difficult gap between paper credentials and actual performance. While board certification and/or college membership are helpful signposts of quality, they are no *guarantee* that a physician is reasonably up-to-date.

There are several ways in which a physician could be forced to keep up. One would be through state licensing powers. While all states require initial test evidence of competency, none requires reexamination for renewal of license. Six states—Iowa, Kansas, Kentucky, Maryland, New Mexico and Vermont—do require evidence of a certain amount of postgraduate study for renewal. A second method would be medical societies insisting on certain standards for maintenance of membership; however, licensed physicians could continue to practice without being members of the appropriate medical society. A third avenue would be for specialty societies to make postgraduate courses and/or reexamination a requirement for continuing membership. While some specialty societies have been very active and even creative in postgraduate education for their members, only two have taken definite steps to require periodic recertification—family practice and surgery.

Of all these, the most likely method to remove incompetents from practice would be mandatory, periodic relicensing—recertification—by examination; such examinations would have to be carefully constructed to accomplish a reasonable purpose—namely, to remove the truly incompetent physician without requiring the average practicing physician to meet standards applicable to the unusual problems of referral and academic centers.

All of this is not meant to suggest that most physicians do not worry about "keeping up." Indeed, the opposite is true in my experience. I have been impressed with how diligently most physicians keep up beyond any requirement to do so—except their own pride and (quite honestly) fear of doing harm to their patients. In my present position in the Department of Continuing Education at Harvard Medical School, I have opportunity to observe the eager learning spirit that still characterizes the majority of physicians. But we must all—physicians and consumers alike— be dedicated to ways of removing incompetents while encouraging the natural desire of most physicians to constantly improve their skills and knowledge.

It would not be unreasonable in evaluating a physician to inquire about continuing education efforts; the office secretary and/or nurse should be able to give such information. Again I remind you of the difficulty of evaluating paper credentials. It is possible to attend courses without really learning, and some of the best learning—journals, informal consultations, etc.—cannot be formally certified ultimately other than by examination. But paper credentials in continuing education do usually indicate a desire for such upgrading, and that's a step in the right direction.

$\mathcal{G}\!$he $\mathcal{S}\!$corecard

At this point we are ready to list doctors by specialty. The commentary is deliberately brief; the main purpose of this listing is to clarify common confusions about names and duties. Comments concerning consumer pitfalls are kept to a minimum; such issues relating to specific specialties will be more fully discussed in the appropriate discussions of Part II.

Allergists

Doctors who treat conditions like hay fever, who try to find out what makes your eyes water and your nose run, who give skin tests and desensitization shots. (See p. 245.)

Most allergy problems are still handled by general practitioners, internists, and pediatricians—all acting as primary care physicians. But some physicians have taken special training or have special interest in this field and have limited their practice. Older allergists were trained mostly by supervised experience; today, however, residency training programs exist.

Many physicians regard allergists as being outside the mainstream of medicine; in part this is because most allergists practice mainly in an office setting and are seldom seen in the hospital. But this feeling is also generated because the work of allergists sometimes seems to be done on an assembly line basis at high cost with limited results.

There are allergists who are extremely competent, very much involved with total medical care, and concerned to individualize their approach to the given patient. Your own primary care physician can probably help you find such a top-notch allergist if you need one.

Dentists

It used to be that all dentists did the same thing. But now even our mouths have become specialized. Actually, the general dentist is still the most common kind of dentist, and he is able to handle the vast majority of dental problems in all age groups. But there are several specialists within the field that you should be aware of:

Endodontists: Dentists who take care of problems with the soft tissue (pulp) in the center of the tooth. They are best known for "root canal" work. Their major theme is tooth preservation; teeth that were readily pulled thirty years ago are now saved by better endodontics. The problem comes when your dentist recommends pulling a tooth: How do you know whether it could be saved? The problem is that you *don't* know—unless you're a dentist yourself— and so you are at the mercy of your dentist's recommendation. For starters, you can ask about the possibility of saving the tooth. If you're not satisfied with the answer you get, you should consider getting an opinion from another dentist. And don't be fooled into thinking that pulling a tooth is cheaper than trying to save it. The initial cost may be less, but the cost of subsequent bridge work may well surpass that of initial root canal treatment.

Oral surgeons: Dentists who concentrate on surgical procedures in the mouth and face. While extractions (such as impacted wisdom teeth) are still the "bread and butter" for oral surgeons, many of them are trained to do extensive surgical work in the facial area—jaw fractures, facial restorations, etc. Who actually does what in a given locality is often a matter of "politics" between the oral surgeons, plastic surgeons, and ENT (ear, nose, and throat) surgeons of a given hospital staff.

Orthodontists: Dentists who straighten teeth. Often some straightening work is essential on children's teeth for adult tooth preservation; other work is largely cosmetic. Fees are high, but, since the process may take two years to complete, per visit costs may not be out of line and usually long-term payment arrangements can be worked out. Adults have become more interested in this kind of corrective work (after they have paid for their kids) and many adult problems can be corrected.

Pedodontists: Dentists who limit their practice to children. Most dental work on children is still done by general dentists. But pedodontists are teaching all of dentistry how to care better for children. One of their most important emphases is proper psychological preparation for dental care—i.e., how not to be afraid of the dentist. Fortunately, most general practice dentists are becoming sensitive to the trauma that can afflict a child in the dental chair.

Periodontists: Dentists who specialize in the care and surgery of the gums. The most important cause of adult tooth loss is periodontal disease—as manifested by red gums which often bleed after brushing. Periodontists specialize in restoring diseased gums; sometimes surgical procedures are necessary to accomplish this.

Again I stress that the general dentist is not a relic of the past. Unlike medicine, general dental information is not impossible to keep up with. However, specialized procedural work (root canals, periodontal surgery, wisdom tooth extractions, straightening appliances, etc.) usually requires the skills of a specialist, and most general dentists will refer to the appropriate specialist.

Dermatologists

Doctors who treat acute adolescent skin problems (acne, blackheads, etc.); adult problems of a similar nature; mysterious rashes which primary care physicians sometimes cannot diagnose; chronic skin ailments like psoriasis, for which no cause or permanent cure has been discovered.

Dermatology as a specialty is quite similar to allergy—a field that used to be covered by primary care physicians totally and still is to large degree. And, like allergists, its practitioners are less involved in hospital medicine.

Like allergists, for complicated cases their expertise can be very useful. The trick is to know when they are really needed; your primary care physician can best advise you. (See page 347.)

General Practitioners

Doctors who ideally should be like a general in terms of the overall view—but who more often are treated like a private in the medical army.

The GP is the most difficult to describe—for many reasons. Historically, his role has gone through many changes and is in a state of great flux today. Half a century ago, physicians were graduated as "physician and surgeon," still a common sign outside a GP's office. That title covers most anything a physician would want to do, and many of them did almost anything—treating heart attacks, setting bones, delivering babies, performing abdominal surgery. Often they performed with remarkable skill and courage. But the increasing difficulty of doing everything well led to the specialization (some would say overspecialization) of today. In some parts of the country, especially in rural areas, the GP still does everything. But in most places his domain has been gradually reduced through restrictions on what he may do in the hospital.

Today, a new trend is beginning. I refer to the "family physician" movement designed to produce a physician better trained in limited areas and more concerned with the total care of the family unit than present specialists. Residencies have been established for family physicians to provide three years of post–medical school training in such areas as internal medicine and pediatrics and the office practice of gynecology, orthopedics, etc. In anticipation of a resurgence of this kind of generalist, the American Academy of General Practice has changed its name to the American Academy of Family Physicians. Also, in 1970 the new American Board of Family Practice conducted its first certifying exams for this "specialty for generalists." (See the later discussion of primary care.)

In the meantime, the oldtime GP must be evaluated carefully. Many are well trained, especially by experience, for what they do, but others are attempting more than their training merits. Often, for routine illness, the tender loving care of the old GP is more than sufficient and may, in fact, be the best medicine. The same cannot be said for critical and complex illnesses.

Internists

Often referred to as the "modern GP," the general internist treats a wide range of nonsurgical problems. In keeping with the trend of specialization, many internists take additional training in one of the subspecialty areas of internal medicine; such subspecialty training is taken as one or more years of "fellowship" after the standard three years of internal medicine residency. The following are the standard areas of internal medicine in which an internist may subspecialize:

Cardiology (diseases of the heart): While most internists receive considerable training in the diagnosis and treatment of heart disorders, many will refer more complicated problems to colleagues with fulltime interest in cardiology. (See page 116.)

Endocrinology (diseases of endocrine organs—i.e., organs which secrete important hormones into the bloodstream—such as the pancreas, the thyroid, etc.): Endocrinologists are acknowledged to be among the most intellectual of physicians—an obvious necessity in this specialty—and a generalization which usually holds true. Most common endocrine disorders (diabetes, thyroid disease, etc.) can be handled by well-trained primary physicians, but the services of an endocrinologist should be considered for any person who has persistent and general ill feeling, since endocrinologists are often superb diagnosticians and may succeed where others have been stumped.

Gastroenterology (diseases of the GI tract—mouth to anus, including stomach, liver, pancreas, intestines): Modern gastroenterologists are trained to do some of the procedures traditionally done by surgeons—endoscopy (putting tubes down via the throat or up via the rectum), biopsy (tissue specimens taken through endoscopy tubes), etc. (See page 159.)

Hematology (diseases of the blood and blood-making tissues): Hematologists are the doctors who become expert at looking at "blood smears" under the microscope. Hematologists usually treat cancers of the blood cells—such as leukemias.

Infectious Disease (ID): Since infectious disease is so common, primary physicians are well exposed to basic information in their training. True ID experts are mostly concerned with unusual bugs and drugs and are called in for the particularly difficult cases of infection—such as FUO's (fevers of unknown origin).

Nephrology (diseases of the kidneys, the rest of the urinary system, and related disorders of metabolism—i.e., electrolyte imbalance, acid-base disturbances, etc.): Nephrologists often work closely with urologists—surgeons who specialize in the urinary system.

Oncology (diseases of abnormal tissue growth—i.e., cancer): With the advent of modern chemotherapy (cancer drugs), most primary physicians cannot provide the expertise required to treat adequately many cancers. The oncologist provides the medical side of such expertise. (See page 155.)

Pulmonary disease (lung disease): As is the case with heart disease, most primary physicians are equipped to handle the common respiratory diseases—pneumonia, chronic lung disease (emphysema), etc. Specialists in pulmonary disease are usually reserved for acute breathing problems (e.g., secondary to trauma) or for terminal (end-stage) breathing difficulties where special machines and knowledge are required.

Rheumatology (diseases of the joints—such as arthritis): Rheumatologists collaborate with orthopedic surgeons in the management of the more severe forms of joint disease. (See page 247.)

Actually, most internists practice general internal medicine but maintain a special interest and expertise in one or more of the above. In teaching hospitals the lines are drawn more tightly; for example, a cardiologist may call in the rheumatologist for a sore toe. (I assume you have heard the terrible joke about the doctor in the Navy who was referred to as a "naval doctor," which prompted a bystander to remark that such superspecialization was carrying things too far.)

Neurologists–Neurosurgeons

Doctors who are concerned with the nervous system— brain, spinal cord, and nerves.

I've lumped these two together because, even though their training is quite different, their concerns are similar, and it is not unusual for them to be together in a group practice. *Neurology* is a branch of internal medicine; most internists are competent to handle basic neurological problems, and most neurologists have had some training in internal medicine. Neurology deals with nonsurgical problems of the nervous system: headaches, Parkinson's disease, multiple sclerosis, etc. *Neurosurgery* is a branch of surgery dealing with surgical problems of the nervous system: head injuries, brain tumors, spinal cord injuries, etc. In many smaller communities without a neurologist, the neurosurgeon also handles nonsurgical problems of the nervous system.

Obstetricians–Gynecologists

Doctors who specialize in conditions affecting the repro- ductive system of women (gynecology) and in the care and delivery of pregnant women (obstetrics).

Years ago, physicians could specialize in either obstetrics or gynecology, and some older physicians consequently limit themselves to one or the other. Today, however, training programs include both and the typical pattern is for the ob-gyn physician to practice both until his later years when he "phases out" obstetrics with its demanding nighttime hours.

Ob-gyn overlaps with several other specialty areas. Many obstetricians become "family physicians" to the women they have delivered, providing annual checkups and advice when needed. Generally, they are not equal to internists on general medical matters, but they may provide interim advice and treatment. Also, many GP's and internists provide basic gynecology care—Pap smears, pelvic exams, etc. Again, they are not the equal of the ob-gyn specialist when it comes to more complex problems but they can usually provide adequate routine care.

Breast cancer, a disease much more common in women than men, is usually the province of the general surgeon, though some gynecologists have been trained in breast surgery. (See page 226.) Most physicians are competent to examine breasts; referral can then be made to a surgeon when necessary.

Ophthalmologists

Physicians who treat eyes with drugs, prescribe glasses, perform surgery on the eyes.

I stress physician because most people confuse this kind of doctor with an *optometrist*, who calls himself a doctor but has no standard medical training. An optometrist is trained to prescribe and prepare glasses; he is not fully trained to recognize and treat all eye problems. In some states, an optometrist is now allowed to use eye drops for examination of the eye. Neither of the above is to be confused with an *optician,* who has even more limited training and does not use the title of doctor. The optician prepares glasses from the prescription of either an ophthalmologist or optometrist.

The critical question is which kind of doctor to go to for glasses—the ophthalmologist, who has considerably more training and expertise in total eye care, or the optometrist, whose expertise is limited to examination for visual acuity and the prescription of glasses. The answer is fairly straightforward: You get what you pay for. The M.D. (ophthalmologist) is usually more expensive, but along with examination for glasses you get the benefit of his full knowledge of eye disease. The optometrist is usually cheaper, and, if the need for glasses is your only problem, you come out paying less. One approach is to use the optometrist for routine problems but to check periodically with an ophthalmologist, especially as you get older and are more likely to encounter other eye problems. (The relationship between ophthalmologists and optometrists has been traditionally strained but is changing more recently to one of guarded cooperation. Changes in various states are allowing the optometrist to enlarge his sphere of activity; some states, for example, now allow the optometrist to examine for glaucoma. You should check the specific situation in your community).

Orthopedic Surgeons (*Orthopedists*)
Doctors who treat bone and joint problems, both surgically and nonsurgically. Simple fractures can be handled by

many general physicians, but in this age of specialization are often referred to an orthopedic surgeon.

Most people with chronic low back pain (oh-my-aching-back) end up with an orthopedist. Disk surgery is performed by both orthopedic surgeons and neurosurgeons. (See page 256.)

Otolaryngologists (*ENT Specialists*)

Doctors who treat ear, nose, and throat (ENT) problems medically and surgically.

Physicians used to specialize in eye, ear, nose, and throat and were called EENT specialists; some older specialists still deal with all four. But eyes have become a separate specialty (ophthalmology), so the younger specialist has lost an E in his title. Radical neck surgery (usually for cancer) may be done by general surgeons, ENT doctors, or plastic surgeons.

Pediatricians

Doctors who take care of children and adolescents. As in internal medicine, subspecialization within pediatrics is the trend—pediatric cardiology, pediatric endocrinology, etc. There is also a trend toward relieving the pediatrician of much of the routine, "well baby" care (shots, feeding schedules, etc.) by the use of specially trained nurses or assistants who handle much of this under the doctor's supervision. Next time you're tempted to call your pediatrician at 2:00 A.M., bear in mind that most physicians agree that these practitioners are the most overworked and underpaid of the specialists.

Psychiatrists

Medical doctors who treat emotional and mental disorders. Psychiatrists have standard medical training (obtaining an M.D.) before three or more years of residency training in the care of mental and emotional disorders. *Clinical Psychologists*—to be distinguished from psychologists who deal with nonclinical matters such as education—differ in having no formal medical training; they obtain a Ph.D instead of an M.D., though much of their training is similar to the post-M.D. training of a psychiatrist. Controversy exists as to whether a psychiatrist needs full medical training even to prescribe drugs or to give shock treatment, which now only psychiatrists—as licensed physicians—can do. The controversy is promoted mainly by mental health workers without an M.D. Psychiatrists are now part of the medical establishment and would like to keep it that way. (See page 286.)

Surgeons

The role of the general surgeon has also changed in recent years. (I suppose no one wants to be a general anything anymore.) The general surgeon of twenty years ago would do all kinds of surgery—scrape out prostates (urology), pin hips (orthopedics), remove lungs (thoracic surgery), etc. Again, in many parts of the country, he still does everything, surgically speaking. But, in the larger cities and especially in teaching hospitals, the general surgeon is restricted to certain parts of the body. Sometimes this is a matter of politics, because the general surgeon may be qualified to do more than he is allowed to do in these hospitals. It should be pointed out that most of the surgical subspecialists are required to take some general surgery

training before their more limited field of surgical training.

Sometimes general surgeons limit themselves to certain
areas of the body (the abdomen, for example) without taking on a special name. Other times, surgeons describe
themselves with special titles. Such special designations
include:

Thoracic surgeon: Surgeons who operate on the chest
(thorax); the lay person sensibly calls them chest surgeons.
Such surgeons have had several years of training beyond
the four years of general surgical training. The chest includes lungs, heart, and esophagus (the food tube from
the throat to the stomach), so these structures are the
major concern of the thoracic surgeon.

Cardiac surgeon: Surgeons who operate on the heart.
Some thoracic surgeons exclude heart surgery from their
area of expertise; others include heart surgery. This designation leaves no doubt.

Cardiovascular surgeon: Surgeons who operate on the
heart and on the blood vessels elsewhere—such as vessels
leading to the brain or the legs or down through the
abdomen. Their training is similar to the thoracic surgeon—several years beyond the required general surgery
training.

Vascular surgeon: General surgeons who have special
training and/or interest in blood vessels outside the chest.

They do not have the additional training of the above three, though they may have had some added training.

Plastic surgeon: A plastic surgeon takes several years of training beyond that of a general surgeon, learning the special techniques of cosmetic surgery, extensive skin grafts, facial injuries, tendon and nerve repair, etc. (See the later section on surgery.)

Proctologist: Surgeons who specialize in "end things" such as hemorrhoids and rectal growths.

Urologist: Surgeons who treat the urinary system (kidneys, bladder, prostate). These physicians work closely with internists specializing in kidney disease, especially in such problems as kidney transplants. Though urologists have become busy doing vasectomies, their most common operation is still removing the enlarged prostates of older men. It is fitting that our survey of the specialties should end with this one in particular, because, as an ancient Greek philosopher once said, "If you can't pee, all else becomes unimportant."

Hospital-Based Specialists
Several other specialties should be mentioned quickly—not because they are unimportant, but because they are usually hospital-based and seen by you only as part of your hospital stay. You have much less choice in dealing with such physicians.

Anesthesiologists put you to sleep in the operating room and, more important, make sure that you wake up; they are also very active (along with pulmonary specialists in internal medicine) in the care of breathing problems, such as those requiring special breathing machines. *Pathologists* are in charge of the laboratories: blood tests, interpreting tissue specimens under the microscopes, autopsies, etc. *Physiatrists* (not to be confused with psychiatrists) are doctors specializing in physical therapy and rehabilitation, an increasingly important part of medical care. *Radiologists* interpret X rays and perform special studies—a GI series, studies of vessels in which dye is injected, etc. All of these hospital-based physicians have specially trained persons who aid in the work of their departments; the training of these technicians has become much more standardized and rigorous in recent years.

Since emergency rooms have become such a prominent part of our health care system, a special word about emergency room physicians is in order. At present, physicians staffing ER's are from all kinds and backgrounds. In most large teaching hospitals, ER's are still largely staffed by "house staff"—interns and residents. Such staffing has obvious advantages (on-the-spot attention, up-to-date experience in emergency procedures, large range of specialty experience readily available, the youthful vigor to attempt treatment of seemingly hopeless situations, etc.) and obvious disadvantages (lack of judgment provided by experience, a sometimes less humane attitude than would be provided by more seasoned physicians, etc.). Some large teaching hospitals are now hiring fulltime, experienced physicians to supervise the work of house staff in the ER.

In many community hospitals ER coverage is provided by members of the medical staff on an assigned, rotational basis; while this may be better than nothing, it is generally unsatisfactory, since not all members of the medical staff have an equal interest or ability in emergency medicine. Increasingly, however, ER's are being staffed by physicians who work fulltime in the ER: they have no outside private practice. Many such fulltimers have come from the ranks of private practice—enticed by the more regular hours of ER practice. Sometimes such physicians come from practice situations where they have been far removed from life-threatening emergencies; the quality of such physicians may be less than desirable if they have not taken special training to correct the lack of such experiences. Unfortunately, standards of practice for emergency physicians have not yet been carefully established by most hospitals.

A healthy development is the fact that more young physicians are choosing emergency medicine as a career. It is just a matter of time before emergency medicine will be a fully recognized specialty; it already has formed a specialty group (the American College of Emergency Physicians), and there are now many two-year programs (post-internship specialty training programs) in emergency medicine being offered throughout the country.

In Addition

Two other kinds of doctors must be mentioned because they are such a prominent part of the health care in this country.

Osteopaths (they put a D.O. at the end of their name) are physicians who have training somewhat similar to that of M.D.'s but with special emphasis on skeletal manipulation. They maintain their own hospitals and specialty training programs, although in many parts of the country they work closely with M.D.'s. There is considerable talk about a merger of M.D.'s and D.O.'s, and it has occurred in some states; nothing on a national scale has happened yet.

Chiropractors are in a class entirely separate from M.D.'s and D.O.'s. Their training is vastly inferior and their practice often suspect from the viewpoint of traditional scientific medicine. I would strongly suggest that you read the following report about chiropractors before going to one: *Independent Practitioners under Medicare: Report to Congress* (Washington, D.C.: Government Printing Office, United States Department of Health, Education and Welfare, 1968; a copy of this report can be obtained by writing or calling the nearest HEW office).

Primary Care

Now that you've read the scorecard, you might well ask, How do I know whom to go to first? The very asking of that question points to the void left by a "family doctor" who is readily available and serves as a guide through medical care. (This book is designed in part to fill that void—but I would be the first to admit that it's only a substitute.)

This problem is usually identified as the "primary care crisis"—meaning the need for health personnel who are readily and economically available for initial screening of health problems and who can intelligently administer further health care of an individual or refer him or her to a specialist when necessary. Traditionally the GP has served as a primary physician; today the internist and pediatrician often fulfill such a role for adults and children, respectively.

It is, however, increasingly difficult to attract doctors into such a role because lower income and status and the difficulty of keeping up with all areas of medical knowledge. As mentioned earlier, there is new impetus to revive the family physician—as reflected in the American Academy of General Practice's change of name to the American Academy of Family Physicians. More important than a change of name is the change in training requirements. Whether this "movement" will actually produce needed numbers of primary physicians is still in doubt. Serious questions remain. Will a public, accustomed to specialty care, accept such a physician for total care? More important, will hospitals long accustomed to limiting the domain of the GP allow this new breed of generalist to reexpand his hospital role commensurate with his training? Will rewards and status be sufficient to attract competent physicians to this three-year training program versus more secure and traditional specialty training?

Another approach to the "crisis" is the development of paramedical personnel—nurse practitioners, physician assistants, etc.—to perform many of the less critical and routine tasks performed by a physician but under his supervision. Most physicians will candidly admit that much of what they do (in some cases, most of what they do) could be competently handled by individuals with less than full medical training. Programs to train such paramedical personnel are now in existence in all parts of the country. As yet, training and performance have not been standardized nationally, but that will come with time. One question involves patient acceptance: Will patients tolerate care from less than a physician? So far the answer seems to be a qualified yes. In short, this is a trend that could provide help for the very real crisis of primary care.

The actual kind of doctor or allied health person who will serve the primary care function for any given person will vary with geography and circumstance. For those living in a highly urbanized area where specialists are the order of the day, the internist for adults and the pediatrician for children will usually serve the primary care function of the fondly remembered GP—able to treat most medical problems, a guide to and judge of other required care, a protector against unnecessary surgery, and a source of general counsel for family problems. For those living in less medically sophisticated areas, general practitioners (or family physicians) may be the cornerstone of medical care. For those in economically deprived areas, clinic facilities may, of necessity, function in this "first line" medical role. In other words, the function of primary care can and will of necessity be filled by several possible resources; sadly, in some instances any resources are difficult to find.

It should be stressed that everyone should strive to establish some kind of primary care relationship (physician, clinic, etc.) *before* a medical problem arises. Amazingly, people will move into a new community and quickly find out about plumbers and car mechanics but not investigate medical resources until an emergency arises.

Changing Practice Patterns

In many areas, patterns of medical practice have changed and are still changing so radically that the choice becomes not which doctor, but which group, clinic, hospital, etc. While the day of the individual practitioner may not be over, most physicians feel that such a form of practice is no longer ideal except in certain situations—isolated areas, highly specialized referral practice, or doctors who can easily limit their hours and who require little coverage when away or sick.

Most doctors, especially primary physicians, find the advantages of group practice too good to pass up—more regular hours, ready coverage, time off for continuing education, and stimulation from constant and close consultation with colleagues. The disadvantages for the physician revolve mainly about the standard difficulties of people getting along in a close relationship (doctors are people, too!). And, while most patients would prefer having just one physician to relate to, they usually recognize the benefits of group practice for them in terms of physicians who are rested and better educated—and one of whom is readily available at any time. There are, however, many different types of "groups." A brief survey may be worthwhile.

Partnership Arrangements

Usually this involves two or more physicians in the same specialty who share an office and work closely together in all phases of practice: office, hospital, night and weekend coverage, etc. Often one of the partners will be "your" doctor in terms of routine office visits, but you must expect to deal with whoever is on call during nights, weekends, and vacations. Such partnership arrangements will often have fancy names and may be incorporated for business purposes (retirement arrangements, etc.).

Clinics

Most people have experienced "clinics" only in the context of large, impersonal hospital settings or as "neighborhood" health programs. Such clinics are often far from ideal in terms of personalized care, but they usually provide competent medical care related to ability to pay—which is something desperately needed by many in our society. One of the more exciting developments in medical care today is the "free clinic" movement where essentially free care is provided for impoverished segments of society by various government or volunteer groups.

The term "clinic" is also sometimes applied to a group practice in which all or most of the specialties are represented—plus many paramedical services such as laboratory,

X ray, physical therapy, etc. Many people think of Mayo or Lahey when they think of "clinics," a complete line of medical services with emphasis on extensive and thorough diagnostic investigation; such clinics are now common in all parts of the United States. Sometimes a "clinic" will be devoted to one disease, such as arthritis or cancer.

HMO's (*Health Maintenance Organizations*)

This phrase originates from government terminology for what is more accurately described as prepaid health insurance arrangements. The basic idea is for an individual or family or larger group to prepay a set sum of money, which guarantees total health care for the given period of time; these arrangements may exempt certain services and cost less accordingly. The basic idea behind such arrangements from a cost viewpoint is that there should be an incentive to maintain health and prevent costly illness—hence the phrase "health maintenance organization"; the less money spent out of the prepaid pot, the more left over to distribute to those providing health care. Thus, one of the most important features of such an arrangement is peer review, the checking of a physician's activity by other physicians to make sure that he does not overcharge or overuse expensive tests and facilities. One of the obvious concerns about this arrangement is that quality will suffer under excessive scrutiny of cost consciousness.

The best known of the HMO plans currently is the California-based Kaiser-Permanente prototype, but the actual mechanics can be worked out in many ways, from the complete hospital clinic setting to a group of physicians who subcontract for any services needed by their subscribers. Because of possible cost savings, there is much interest at the government level in this kind of medical arrangement, but many feel that important questions of cost, incentive, and quality remain to be answered.

Foundations

This term usually designates a medical society (local, county, or state) that has formed an organization to deal with payments to physicians in its area. It represents a quasi-union to present a united way to deal with payers of medical care—individuals, insurance companies, Medicaid, etc. Many foundations have prepayment contracts and thus incorporate the strong peer review features which have been described earlier.

If all this suggests that the logistics of health care are in a state of upheaval, that should come as no surprise: You read about it every day.

Choosing a Doctor

We are now in a position to summarize much of what has been said thus far—and add a few more practical points concerning the choice of a doctor. The fact that the majority of physicians are competent should not keep you from trying to avoid the bad apple before taking a bite and finding out the hard way. Even though medical practice is much more standardized than it was fifty years ago, there is still a significant difference among physicians. And, unlike airline pilots, once licensed, a physician can practice without periodic checking of his skills in any official way. Here, then, is a checklist of suggestions:

1. Choose a physician active in a good hospital. As indicated earlier, the best kind of control exerted on physicians today is via their peers in the hospital. It is not perfect, but it is the best thing going. You'll be reading a lot about *peer review* in the future; the concept is good (for all professions), though the mechanics are, at times, difficult.

2. Inquire very specifically about a physician's training and expertise. You may be embarrassed to ask the physician himself, but you can certainly inquire through other sources—his office, the local or state medical society, or the hospital where he practices.

3. Don't be afraid to shop around a little. I am not encouraging the kind of doctor-hopping that all physicians are familiar with—the continual running from one doctor to another. But you are not legally married to a physician you are unhappy with; discreet changes can be made. Sometimes dissatisfaction is a simple matter of personality conflict, which can originate on either side—or both. And it is perfectly reasonable to get another opinion when serious treatment, such as major surgery, is recommended. (See page 51.)

4. Evaluate carefully the advice of friends and neighbors. Sometimes this advice can be very valuable—if, for example, it comes from a real insider, such as a nurse or a hospital technician who works closely with physicians. But sometimes advice is based purely on a limited reaction to the personality of a physician—which is important, but not as important as the knowledge that's between his ears.

5. Do a little self-analysis as part of the choice process. Are you the kind of person who requires a doctor with a high "patience quotient"—willing and available to answer and explain? Or do you prefer the person of few words who acts with silent authority?

6. Geographical convenience should not be underestimated. If your time or transportation are limited, don't get involved with a clinic miles away when a competent physician is available right in your com-

munity. Primary care physicians (internists, pediatricians, family physicians) must be readily available to be valuable.

7. Remember that the age of a physician *might* be important. For example, if you are young and looking for a long-range association with a primary care physician, it would seem best to look for a younger doctor. Also, an older doctor may not be as available or up-to-date as a doctor just starting out. On the other hand, experience can be a valuable asset in difficult situations. Age and its ramifications for you, must be considered when making a choice.

8. Finally, if you are moving and you are satisfied with your present physician, ask him to recommend someone in the area you are moving to. Often he will have contacts elsewhere or can find out about someone suitable for you. You will not be bound by his recommendations, but it provides a start in your search.

The Question of Surgery

For the person to whom surgery has been recommended, two critical questions immediately surface: Is this surgery necessary? Is this surgeon competent? In an emergency situation, such as massive bleeding from the stomach, there is little time to answer such questions. But most surgery is "elective"—i.e., there is time to consider such questions without the threat of death intervening.

Is It Necessary?

The answer to this question requires some investigating. This can be done in several ways:

1. At the very least, a second opinion could be elicited whenever major surgery is recommended. This can be done while in the hospital by asking your primary physician (if you have one) to arrange a second surgical opinion. If you are out of the hospital, a second opin-

ion is easily arranged. I am not saying that a second opinion must *always* be sought, but, if major surgery is being recommended by a surgeon you do not know or have no knowledge of, hold off making a decision until you can check further.

2. Don't hesitate to do a little reading in standard medical sources. I know some of my colleagues will argue with this, but I am convinced that most people who have basic intelligence can gain valuable medical information by reading. (See the bibliography at the end of this book.)

3. Be sure to ask the recommending surgeon to detail the options and risks. What will happen if you don't have the surgery? What might happen if you do? Don't expect any reputable surgeon to give absolute guarantees or fixed odds. But he should be prepared to defend the logic of his recommendation. The age is long past when you have to take such verdicts on faith.

All of this is to recognize that unnecessary surgery does occur—not as much as some would suggest, but enough to make careful investigation worthwhile. In Part II, I will deal with some specific areas in which unnecessary surgery commonly occurs.

Is the Surgeon Competent?

This question is more difficult. The fact of the matter is that there is a significant difference between board-certified surgeons as judged according to the following criteria:

1. *Clinical judgment.* This phrase covers ability outside the operating room—deciding when to operate, han-

dling complications, etc. There are surgeons who are skilled mainly in the operating room.

2. *Technical ability.* This refers to whether a surgeon has "good hands" or "bad hands"—meaning, of course, the way he actually performs surgery. While this is obviously important, it is not the total story.

3. *Intestinal Fortitude.* "Guts" is the best word I can think of to describe this all-important quality in a surgeon. I am referring to what it is that separates the men from the boys in the heat of fire—either during or after a difficult operation. In part, guts involves willingness to be available whenever a problem arises; it also involves a degree of dedication; and, finally, it involves how quickly one gives up in a seemingly hopeless situation.

While physicians other than board-certified surgeons may be perfectly adequate to handle minor surgical problems (lacerations, minor skin abnormalities, etc.), major surgery (abdominal, chest, vascular, etc.) should not be done by persons with less than the training of a board-certified surgeon. I will get some argument on this one from a few physicians, but the vast majority will agree with me.

The fact of the matter is that in most cases the surgeon is selected by a referring physician—usually the primary care physician who has been responsible for the case up to the point where surgery is recommended. If you have confidence in your primary care physician (internist, pediatrician, GP, family doctor), then you may be willing to let him "pick" a surgeon for you. Many primary care physicians work in association with certain surgeons and will obviously recommend those surgeons. You are *not* bound to accept the recommendation of your primary care physician. If you have good reason to want another surgeon or to want time to check around, you have every right to so ask. If your primary care physician gets upset about that, that's his problem—not yours. But, again, if you have confidence in the primary care physician you are dealing with, you will probably be as well off accepting his choice of a surgeon as trying to investigate matters on your own.

Plastic Surgery

A special word about plastic surgery is in order, since the kind of work the plastic surgeon does is probably one of the most misunderstood in medicine. Often the plastic surgeon is misused due to such misunderstandings. And, since their price is usually high, it is worth understanding when they should be called upon.

The plastic surgeon is first trained as a general surgeon before beginning a further two to three years in the special techniques of nerve repair, tendon repair, hand surgery, burn therapy, facial reconstruction, etc. Most plastic surgeons that I have talked to "off the record" agree that the prolonged training in general surgery is unnecessary, since the plastic surgeon will almost never be involved with most areas of general surgery again; it is, quite frankly, a matter of "union" requirements—and an excellent way of keeping numbers limited and the quality high.

Such prolonged training, however, adds to the mystique and prices of the plastic surgeon. That mystique includes the idea that, unless a laceration is repaired by plastic surgeons using "plastic techniques," the scar will be worse than otherwise. The result, in our specialty-oriented society, is a young mother who insists on a plastic surgeon for the one-inch cut on her child's leg.

The fact is that any experienced physician can repair simple lacerations according to so-called "plastic technique"—which in this case means careful attention to minimize scarring. (No physician in his right mind will promise "no scar"—though with careful repair and good care by the patient that may be the end result.) Thus, when your child gets a simple laceration of the face, you should question your own doctor or the physician in the emergency room as to the need for a plastic surgeon.

So far I have minimized the necessity of plastic surgeons in simple, routine lacerations. Now I come to praise them —for the kind of expertise they do have in more complicated problems relating to both cosmetic surgical repair (to improve the looks) and traumatic surgical repair (necessary as the result of an accident). I have seen some fantastic surgery done by creative and skillful plastic surgeons that is worth every penny they have charged. In such difficult situations, a well-trained and experienced plastic surgeon can be worth his weight in gold.

The problem is that in plastic surgery, as in every field of medicine, some practitioners are better than others. And, in the difficult case, it pays to seek out the better ones. The other problem is that plastic surgery fees are almost always high—in some cases entirely justifiably so, but in many other cases not so. And, since most elective plastic surgery is not covered by insurance, you should talk turkey about fees with a plastic surgeon before proceeding with elective surgery. If you truly cannot afford the work, say so, explain your situation, and ask for advice as to how to proceed; the surgeon may be willing to modify his usual fee or direct you to a clinic situation which can provide good work at lower cost.

By now you have probably gathered that I am not in great sympathy with the "cosmetic" movement of our age

—particularly the "face-lift" assembly lines for the aging wealthy. As long as there is money to pay, there will be doctors willing to operate. But I would like to see that time and talent spent on more legitimate medical needs. I know that's unrealistic—but I present this as one of my biases.

The Surgical Environment

As important as the surgeon is, the total surgical environment of the hospital is almost equally as important. Foremost in this "environment" is the anesthesiology department. This department, besides being responsible for the administration of anesthesia during surgery, usually sets the standards for the way in which the operating room and recovery room are run. Anesthesiologists are doctors who have specialized in this field; anesthetists are nonphysicians (usually specially trained nurses) who give anesthesia under the direction of a doctor. Sometimes doctors work parttime or fulltime in giving anesthesia without having had formal residency training; fortunately, that practice is much less common today than twenty years ago.

Frankly, it is almost impossible for an outsider to assess accurately the surgical environment of a hospital. You can, however, ask your surgeon about what to expect: who will give the anesthesia, who will be responsible for your recovery from surgery, etc. And you should *never* have an operation (except under emergency circumstances) without first being visited by a member of the department of anesthesiology; this person should examine you, describe what is going to happen, and answer any questions you might have.

The question of *informed consent* is one of the most

controversial and complex issues in all of medicine and particularly in the performance of surgery and other procedures that carry risk. Basically, the idea of informed consent is what the words suggest—i.e., you should be asked to give consent (sign the paper approving what the doctors are going to do) only after you have been adequately informed about the pros and cons of the surgery or procedure being proposed. The problem here is obvious: What is meant by "adequate information"? Some people have interpreted *adequate* to mean *everything* (that is, that you should be informed of everything that has ever been written or known about the procedure in question). Others point out that such completeness is impossible and impractical. Some doctors insist that, if certain patients are told about some of the risks, they will become so upset that they will turn down an operation which they really do need. I don't pretend to be able to answer this one— when lawyers and doctors far more experienced than I cannot agree on what constitutes "informed consent." I can tell you, however, that you have a legal right to know everything you *want* to know about a treatment that is being proposed for you. At the very least, you should ask about the major risks involved versus the benefits to be expected.

Finally, a word about high-risk surgery, such as open heart surgery. Such surgical procedures are best done in hospitals and by surgeons who do them frequently. Just how often a surgeon and hospital need to do a given operation to be good at it is difficult to say. When high-risk surgery is required, large teaching hospitals generally offer the best total surgical environment.

Doctors and Money

This section presents an issue much on the minds of all of us—physicians and consumers alike. I offer it as a brief attempt to give some perspective for your future thought.

At the outset, it should be said that doctors account for a relatively small part of total health costs in this country. It is, however, the part that is most visible and identifiable: A bill from your doctor (especially for routine office visits) stands out in black and white and is often not covered by insurance. It's much easier to complain about a person than about the vague "health care industry."

Add a couple of other considerations sometimes not thought of. First, it seems downright unfair to pay for something like illness, which is annoying at best, devastating at worst—and which we certainly didn't ask for. It's one thing to moan about paying for repairs on our new car; for that, however, we at least are partly responsible since we decided to buy it in the first place. But illness is on nobody's menu of life. (By the way: Doctors often fail to appreciate the annoyance of paying for illness, since they usually provide "professional courtesy" for each other for costs not covered by insurance.)

A second consideration: Most people harbor a kind of secret resentment toward physicians in general—though they usually hold their own doctor in high regard. And I think this resentment is understandable, though not logical. After all, a physician seemingly has his cake and can eat it too: He or she lives an apparently exciting life, is well regarded—and gets well paid to boot. So the Cadillac with M.D. on the license plates is resented—but other Cadillacs on the road can pass by and not be given a second thought. Or people talk about all the doctors who belong to the Country Club, forgetting the insurance executives, construction company owners, et al., who belong. Another example: I heard very little criticism of the lawyers who charged former President Nixon hundreds of thousands of dollars for legal fees; it was often described as "a fact of life." But, had his doctors submitted a bill for anything near that amount, a large public outcry would have been likely.

One more consideration before I switch to the other side of the fence: Until quite recently, doctors-in-training lived a near-poverty existence for many years, an existence made no easier by observing their college classmates out earning a good living. So when, six to twelve years after college, they do get out into the "real world," they literally and figuratively try to make up for lost financial time— paying off debts and gratifying long repressed consumer urges that peers had been satisfying for years. More recently, doctors-in-training (interns and residents) have been more fairly compensated; this may moderate the desire to make up for lost time.

Most people, when confronted with cold logic, are ready to agree that physicians—given the years of training, hours worked, and responsibilities assumed—deserve a very good income. But we humans more often think with emotion rather than cold logic. I am trying to suggest some of the emotional factors that color our thinking about physicians and money. (For that matter, there is very little logic in most of the compensation patterns of our society, where a schoolteacher to whom we entrust our children for so much of their young lives makes $10,000 a year and an athlete is rewarded with millions—not to mention inherited wealth.)

But, given the logic of physicians earning well-above-average incomes, there are some doctor–money matters that bother me—and that all of us, as medical consumers, should be aware of.

In my estimation, most prominent among these concerns is the inequity of incomes among various specialties. There often seems to be little relationship between what a physician does and how he is paid. For example, the hard-working pediatrician, putting in long hours and taking many night calls, makes much less than the surgical subspecialist who works half the time and has few night calls. Even within the surgical field, fee schedules often defy reason. For example, a difficult gall bladder operation with demanding followup care may be "worth" $400, while a relatively simple prostate operation with minimal post-op care may "bring" $600.

I'll share an example from my own circle of acquaintances. A young woman had a rather serious kidney problem, for which she was hospitalized in a prominent university hospital. The internist—who supervised her case, gave it considerable time and effort over a five-day period, and was ultimately responsible for the difficult treatment decisions—was allowed by Blue Shield $150 for his efforts. The urologist—who spent some twenty minutes in a surgical open biopsy—was allowed $400. As has often been said, ours is a society that rewards doers—not thinkers.

At this point I should take a minute to explain "fee schedules." Most of the things physicians do are charged for according to fee schedules that have been established by third-party payers—insurance companies and the government, primarily. Actually, these fee schedules have been largely determined by committees of doctors. There have been two problems with the development of these fee schedules. First, many of these committees setting up fee schedules have been dominated by surgeons who, not surprisingly, have suggested that their work is more important and difficult than the work of other physicians. No one would argue that open heart surgery is "worth" more than a routine physical exam—though some would suggest that a wise diagnostician who detects a correctable problem at an early stage can be as valuable as a surgeon who functions as a highly skilled technician. What most physicians and, I think, objective outside observers would argue for is reevaluation of fee schedules based on factors of training, time, difficulty, etc. As the situation now stands, the inequities of current fee schedules are accepted under the euphemistic phrase "usual and customary"—meaning that "the way things are is the way they are going to be." Second, it is admittedly difficult to quantify "thought" and "judgment" skills. It is much easier to put a price tag on a procedure. My answer to this problem is this: Let's admit that this is a problem, but let us not allow that admission to keep us from attempting to reevaluate physician compensation patterns.

I should make it absolutely clear that I am not arguing for the lowering of all physicians' incomes; in my estimation some make too much for what they do and many others (especially conscientious primary care physicians) make too little for their training and efforts when compared to what others in our society make for much less effort and responsibility. What I am arguing for is a reevaluation of the inequities that currently exist among physicians—including hospital-based physicians who often work on a "percentage" basis that bears little relationship to what they actually do. In fact, a recent survey (by a company called Kearney Management Consultants) indicated that over half of both pathologists and radiologists working in hospitals of 100 to 249 beds make more than $110,000 per year. That is much more than most primary care physicians—and without most of the night and weekend responsibilities of other doctors.

Apart from the irritation produced *within* the medical community by such inequities, especially toward large sums for relatively simple surgical procedures, this matter should be of concern to medical consumers because it has an effect on the interest in primary care by young physicians. Human nature being what it is, a choice between working seventy hours a week as a pediatrician for one-half the income of a surgical subspecialist working only thirty-five hours will become for some young physicians a choice based on personal comfort rather than on true personal interest or the actual needs of society.

Another concern is the question of "fee-for-service." Doctors are criticized for attempting to preserve fee-for-service versus allegedly more economical salaried arrangements. The real issue, in my estimation, should be the maintenance of incentive. If physicians become nine-to-five professionals, stripped by working arrangements of personal relationship to or concern about a given patient, I am convinced that the quality of care will suffer. I would be the first to support other arrangements that can provide the same incentive, relationship, responsibility that fee-for-service does—but I have as yet to be convinced that a good substitute exists. In other words, I think there will always have to be some kind of financial incentive; I wish it weren't necessarily so, but this is Earth, not Heaven where money supposedly will no longer talk. I say this even though I personally am happy as a salaried physician.

There are physicians who are greedy, overcharging discredits to the profession. They are in a minority, but they stick out like sore thumbs. They irritate the rest of the profession just as they do the public. But there is little any of us can do about them, as long as there are people who are willing to pay their prices in a free enterprise society. Plastic surgeons charging large fees for cosmetic surgery seem to have no trouble finding rich patients who will pay their price. And as long as this situation exists such doctors will exist.

Finally, a quick word about how to handle what you think is an excessive fee. Again, I remind you that most fees—especially for procedures covered by insurance—are predetermined by schedules that most physicians simply refer to in making out their bills. As mentioned above, these schedules are sometimes very illogical, but, until they are changed by third-party carriers, doctors will continue to use them. However, some doctors will charge even more for reasons they think are justified—their reputation, the special nature of the case, etc. If you think a given fee is unreasonable in terms of the doctor's training and what was done, you should proceed as follows:

First, before making a federal case of it, talk directly to the doctor or his office staff. Many times, an honest mistake was made and is easily corrected. Often, an explanation of the given situation will be satisfactory. And, quite frankly, most doctors will lower the fee in a dispute rather than take the time and effort to follow the dispute into channels of arbitration. Second, if the above measures fail, take your concern to the local and/or state medical society. Such organizations now have "grievance" committees which look into fee disputes; they are anxious to avoid the bad publicity of fee gouging and will be very receptive to your complaint. If your complaint is legitimate, they will put pressure on the physician to lower his fee. And, while this pressure does not have the force of a court order, a physician would have an almost impossible time collecting more than such a committee recommends. The point is that you do have recourse for the uncommon but troublesome unreasonable fee.

When to See a Doctor

This section deals with specific symptoms and situations. Right now, I would like to discuss three general categories of decisions concerning medical care.

The Annual Exam

Many physicians, and I am among them, feel that the *traditional* "annual physical" has been overpromoted. Notice that I emphasize that it is the traditional version of the annual exam I object to—the patient without a specific problem or complaint going to the doctor or clinic for a head-to-toe check. Most physicians would agree that, in the absence of any specific complaint, chronic problem, or family history that needs checking, the annual exam is usually unrewarding.

Obviously one should see a physician *whenever* a serious sign of disease arises; putting off doing something about the discovery of "a little blood in the stools" until you get

time for "a good checkup" is sheer foolishness. And there
are certain preventive measures which should be done on
a regular basis, including:

1. *Blood pressure check:* It is now clear that control of
   even mild elevation in blood pressure pays off. And
   the problem is that high blood pressure usually causes
   no symptoms until later in the game. You should arrange for such a check by anyone who can take blood
   pressure at least once a year. (A good cuff on the arm
   might pay off.) (See page 309.)

2. *Pap smear:* I am amazed at how many women still do
   not have this done at least once a year. The test is
   simple, cheap, and very effective at detecting early
   cervical cancer—and cervical cancer which can be cured
   in almost 100 percent of cases *if* detected early. There
   have been experiments with "home kits" to accomplish
   the same screening for cervical cancer, but as yet they
   are not as effective as the traditional Pap smear. (See
   page 234.)

3. *Breast exam:* Again, I am amazed how many women
   still do not self-examine the breasts once a month; for
   those still menstruating, six to eight days after the flow
   has stopped is the best time. Both visual inspection
   and systematic palpation (touching) of the breasts in
   several positions are required. (See page 223.)

4. *Glaucoma testing:* Ideally, all physical examinations in
   an adult should include examination with a tonometer
   —a device placed on the eye to check for increased
   pressure in the eye. Most forms of glaucoma have a
   slow and insidious onset and can be detected only by
   such pressure testing. Adults are advised to take advantage of glaucoma testing clinics when available.
   (See page 293.)

5. *Blood testing for cholesterol and triglycerides:* At least one check of these "blood fats" rather early in life would be wise in terms of what we think we know about heart disease. If elevated, they should be treated and followed. If normal, one need not repeat the tests very often; every five years is sufficient. Remember that at least twelve hours of no eating and drinking before the tests is required for accurate results. (See page 130.)

6. *Blood sugar:* While not necessary on a routine basis, a blood sugar check occasionally—especially as one grows older—is in order. In anyone with a family history of diabetes it should be done with regularity. (See page 273.)

You might wonder why I have left the chest X ray off the above list. It is an excellent way of looking at the heart and lungs (and other chest structures) when there are symptoms. But the payoff from routine annual screening in the absence of symptoms has been questioned in recent years—except in certain high-risk groups. I'm not specifically advising against chest X rays, but I can't honestly promote them either.

The EKG (heart tracing) is in the same category. While it would be wise for everyone over forty to have at least one EKG as a kind of baseline (and to keep a record of the results), to promote it on an annual basis in the absence of complaints would be misleading.

All of this is not to say that a routine exam cannot be worthwhile. Indeed, as we grow older, a periodic checkup becomes more important. In fact, as we grow older we are more likely to develop specific problems requiring us to see the doctor. But in the absence of specific problems, the routine checkup for young, healthy people is not the best way to spend our limited medical time or money.

The Emergency

A true emergency (sudden, excruciating chest pain or massive vomiting of blood) is one time you should *not* call the doctor; you shouldn't waste even the minutes it might take to reach a doctor. Instead, you should arrange to get to the nearest emergency room as soon as possible. Preferably, you should go to the hospital where your doctor practices, and you may want to have someone notify his office or answering service that you are on the way to the hospital. *But you should not waste time trying to get him or wait for him to call back.* Despite all its faults, the emergency room is one place open twenty-four hours a day where a medical problem usually will receive prompt and competent care and, when necessary, serve as an efficient route to hospitalization.

House Calls

Most people gripe about the current rarity of the house call, because the house call symbolizes for them so much of what they miss from the "good old days" in general and the "good old family doctor" in particular: personal attention and concern at any hour. (Let's face it, TLC—tender loving care—is tough to find anywhere in our modern, depersonalized society.) But most people usually understand two very good reasons why house calls are seldom made anymore:

Efficiency: A doctor can see several patients in the office or the hospital in the time it takes him to make an isolated house call. In this age of doctor shortage this is an important consideration.

Effectiveness: Aside from TLC (which I don't mean to minimize) there is not much the physician has to offer in the home. If the condition is really serious, the hospital, where diagnostic and treatment equipment is readily available, is a much better place to meet the physician.

Having said this, I will also say that we in the medical profession have not done our full duty to provide house calls where they are legitimate—namely, for the disabled person or invalid who needs only maintenance care and who finds it difficult to get out of the home. Such persons usually do not need the attention of a physician, but it should be our responsibility to see that visiting nurses (or their equivalent) are provided.

How a Doctor Thinks

Volumes have been written about the complex interpersonal dynamics of the physician–patient relationship, but I'm going to deal at a more practical level and attempt to give you some insight as to what the modus operandi of the typical physician is like—and what its implications are for you. Again I remind you (as I did in the introduction) that this entire book—and especially the material in this section—is geared to those in our society fortunate enough to be able to choose and evaluate medical care. For many in our country, stuck in the pit of poverty or ignorance, the kinds of considerations I am about to present are far removed from the much more basic problem of finding *any* kind of medical care.

The Physician as Computer–Detective

For many medical consumers, the physician represents a kind of human computer. The patient offers input data in providing information to the doctor by answers to questions, the results of tests, and the sights and sounds and sensations of the physical exam. Out come the answers as to what's wrong, it is hoped, and, more important, what to do about it.

The physician looks upon the process as would a detective. As soon as the patient provides a clue or clues (which often occurs before a word is uttered), the physician becomes a snoop on the trail of "what's a causin'-it" (versus "whodunit"). The better and more experienced the physician, the more skilled he is at gathering and interpreting evidence; like a good detective, many physicians have an exquisitely developed sixth sense which puts them on the trail almost immediately. (Incidentally, the analogies of computer and detective highlight two views of the physician: One recognizes that much of what is done by a physician can be done by machines, while the other recognizes that a machine will never replace the role of judgment so important in a good physician.)

The search is usually conducted under the influence of several unwritten "laws" which have become deeply ingrained during the long years of medical training. One law is often referred to in medical school as "Sutton's Law"—named after the famous bankrobber Willie Sutton, who, when asked why he robbed banks said, "Because that's where the money is." So the physician is reminded to think of the obvious cause, because that's most likely to be the culprit. For example, a woman of child-bearing age who has missed several periods is most likely pregnant; more esoteric endocrine causes must be considered but not to the exclusion of the obvious. (Another way of putting this: If you hear hoofbeats during the night, think of horses and not zebras—unless you live in Africa.)

A second law is that of the pessimist: Always think of

the worst. This usually provides a dilemma for the physician, as I will relate, because to rule out the worst with certainty often means an extensive and expensive investigation (or "workup," as doctors call it) which will likely turn out negative. But the conscientious physician is always haunted by the responsibility not to miss something important.

A third law is that of the optimist: Always think of something you can correct. The natural hope of both patient and physician is that something treatable can be found as cause of the problem; it is tragic to overlook such possibilities. For example, even for a person with apparently incurable lung cancer, there may be complicating or secondary lung infections which can be treated, thereby providing the patient with a more comfortable existence.

The Art of Medicine

The real art of medicine comes in balancing the apparently contradictory concerns of the above "laws"—and others like them. This is what judgment, wisdom, and experience are all about—how to steer a course between competing considerations that will be in the best total interests of the patient and "do no harm." Quite frankly, the difficult decisions are often influenced by nonmedical considerations, among which are the following:

Legal concerns: I hesitate to put it first on the list, but I honestly feel that this is as important a nonmedical consideration as any. There is no question that many tests are ordered "just to be on the safe side." Most of these tests are not harmful, so little is lost except time and money. Indeed, if the decision involves a more dangerous test or operation, then the consideration to "play it safe" might favor *not* doing something that could be life-saving. (Fortunately, this kind of ultimate choice is relatively uncommon or most physicians would go mad under the burden.)

The whole question of malpractice suits is beyond the scope of this treatise, but it is a question that society as a whole and the legal and medical professions in particular must resolve so that medical care is not compromised by legal considerations. Don't misunderstand me: I am all for just compensation for misfortune, let alone malpractice, and the proper scrutiny of medical care on the patient's behalf is absolutely essential. What I and many physicians object to is the great ease with which unfounded charges are given the status of a lawsuit, causing great embarrassment to physicians and considerable cost to society. The fact is that, of all claims brought against physicians, only a very small percent are successful; there should be a more efficient and less sensational way of justly compensating those injured by medical care.

Social status: I would be less than candid if I did not put this on the list. There is no question that in many borderline situations the person with means and connections will get the extensive workup while the person of lesser status will not. Inequality of opportunity sadly pervades all of our society, including medical care. Presidents get better care than paupers. Having made this indictment of our health care system, I will qualify it by saying that in my experience a patient's lack of money has seldom prevented what is really necessary from ultimately being done, though necessary arrangements may take time and more than usual effort.

One important question is the alleged abuse of the poor and ignorant for purposes of training and research. Again, a thorough exploration of this important question is much beyond this discussion. Ultimately, in medicine, as in all life, we become mutually dependent on each other's integrity—whether politician, or salesman, or physician. I can honestly say, however, that I have seen *very little* such abuse in my own medical experience in several medical settings; when "abuse" has existed, it has been more related to the immediate situation rather than to racial or social considerations. For example, the "drunk" or "drug addict" may be mistreated, but that happens quite apart from his skin color or the thickness of his wallet.

Patient anxiety: This factor cannot be overemphasized. Many skull X rays have been ordered to appease anxious parents, even though the physician knows clearly that no serious head injury is present. In the profession we speak of the "therapeutic test," meaning that the doing of the test will itself make the patient feel better and reassure him that nothing is wrong. Sometimes we physicians try to explain why a test is not necessary, but often we give in to the obvious concern that "everything possible be done."

This factor also strongly affects the decision to treat. Physicians soon learn that some people will simply not be happy until something is done to them or for them. For example, much vitamin B-12 has been given for patient satisfaction, not medical necessity; at least no harm is done. But the same cannot be said of the enormous amounts of unnecessary penicillin which have been given for viral conditions in which antibiotics are not effective;

unlike the vitamin shot, the penicillin shot is not without danger in terms of immediate or future reactions. The days of Uncle John's Snake Oil are not entirely gone.

The Actual Encounter

Now, what should all of the above mean to you when you see a doctor? First, come prepared with as much useful information for the "computer" as possible—past history, medications, etc. Like all computers, the physician is dependent on input.

Second, don't be afraid to ask questions concerning what's happening inside the "computer's" brain. Be suspicious of the physician who becomes unduly angered by legitimate inquiry. Obviously anyone will become annoyed at being continually challenged in his area of expertise, but no decent physician should be put off by sincere concern to know what is going on. (Do remember that physicians are human in the same ways you are—they fight with their wives or husbands, worry about their kids. You can hit them at a bad moment, as you can any other member of the human race.)

And, finally, appreciate the physician who tries to avoid unnecessary tests and treatment. Don't be afraid to ask him what he would do in the same circumstances for a member of his own family; that's a pretty good standard to follow. The compassionate computer is one that is not obligated to act in a certain way but can adapt to the real situation at hand.

Common *Medical* Problems

Now that you know something about choosing health care, we can focus on specific medical problems. (I will presume that you have read Part I and are familiar with its terminology—particularly the listing of specialists.) The "mini-discussions" in this part are not intended to be comprehensive for a given problem. Rather, they are intended to zero in on what I consider to be the essential information that should be known and used by everyone. Obviously there will be specific variations in each individual situation; you should never follow the advice of this or any other book against your own better instincts. When in doubt, *check it out.*

Viewed in another manner, these mini-discussions attempt to cut through the mass of medical information available to the general public and highlight issues of controversy and/or prevention. There is a certain danger in taking a position on some of these issues because the information can change literally overnight. But I find that it is the confusion of opinions that is often the most frustrating part of choosing health care. So, where it is reasonably legitimate to do so, I have taken a stand.

Throughout these discussions, I use the phrase "good evidence." Since I have deliberately avoided the use of backup data in the interest of readability, I should explain what I consider to be "good evidence." "Good evidence" in medical science requires the following approach. As a minimum, such information must be published in a reputable manner so that other scientists can examine the information and attempt to confirm (reproduce) the reported results. Ideally, clinical information regarding new methods of diagnosis and treatment should come from RCT's—randomized clinical trials. While there is considerable discussion as to the exact mechanics of such trials, the basic idea is to remove personal bias from the study so that the information obtained will be as objective as possible. In order to do this, both the "observer" (the person doing the study) and the "observed" (the persons being studied) must be kept from knowing which alternative (the new or the "control") is being tested; thus the name "double blind" is often applied to such studies. There is an enormous amount of medical "information" that has not been subjected to these standards. The most suspect information is so-called "anecdotal" information—i.e., information based on the personal experience of a given doctor or patient. While such information may indeed turn out to be valid when subjected to the kinds of studies just described, it cannot honestly be promoted for general consumption until that has been done. When I refer to "good evidence," then, I am talking about the kind of evidence that has been substantiated by appropriate studies and has been published for examination by others.

Another phrase used widely in this part of the book needs explanation, namely the phrase "a good primary care physician." As discussed in greater detail in Part I, obtaining good primary care is the cornerstone to any program of medical care. Primary care, as defined earlier, means "health personnel who are readily and economically available for initial screening of health problems and who can intelligently provide and direct the further health care of an individual." This is obviously the function performed by the competent GP or family doctor of previous times. Today this function is often divided between internists for adults and pediatricians for children. In many communities, the GP or newer-model family doctor still provides most primary care. In inner-city areas, the clinic of the large teaching hospital often serves this function, sometimes in a manner that leaves much to be desired in terms of personal considerations. Thus, when I use the phrase "good primary care physician" I mean any source of competent primary care, including qualified clinics, which may use paramedical personnel under careful supervision. It is critical for each individual and/or family to establish some primary care medical relationship before it is actually needed in the moment of illness.

Now a word about the organization of this part: I have been torn between two alternatives: putting all the discussions into alphabetical order or grouping them according to a common "theme" or body part. I have finally decided to compromise and do some of both. Thus, the first eight sections (Emergencies, Heart Disease, Lung Disease, Cancer, Gastrointestinal Disease, Infectious Disease, Nutrition, Women's Health Problems) contain material that is introductory or that should be grouped together. The last section contains discussions that are grouped in strictly alphabetical order. My hope is that you will read all of this material straight through, and it is occasionally assumed that you have read previous sections; if you want to locate a particular topic quickly, you should use the index.

Finally, I would urge you take advantage of the many sources of medical consumer information. While there may be oversimplification and even misinformation in some of these popular media reports, at least you will be alerted to current issues in medical diagnosis and treatment and you can then engage in more meaningful dialogue with those who provide your health care. You should never be afraid to ask questions; since it's your body, time, and money, you have every right to expect reasonable answers to your questions. (See the bibliography at end of book.)

Emergencies

This first section of Part II deals with emergencies that anyone might be exposed to, beginning with those that are often life-threatening and proceeding to others that are usually less serious. It is my firm conviction that *anyone* should be able to handle the situations discussed in this section.

1

Emergencies

This section deals with those kinds of situations where you don't have time to "look it up" in the first-aid manual or any other source of information. Maybe the best word to use to describe the situation I am talking about is "collapse." This word covers those situations in which a person actually falls to the ground or is found in an apparent state of unconsciousness. Such occasions require immediate judgment and/or action. Though there is no fourteen-karat substitute for training and experience, I will try to give some guidelines which could be helpful.

The most important thing to do initially if you are with, or come upon, someone who has collapsed is to remain calm and take *a few well-chosen seconds* to assess the situation. I can hear your protests: That's easier said than done—especially for someone who has had no experience in emergency situations. Stick with me, because it's precisely for that "someone who has had no experience" that I am writing this section.

It is essential that you understand that there are only

two functions that are immediately life-threatening when absent—*breathing* and *circulation*. Put immediately into practical terms, this means that if you can *feel a breath* and *feel a pulse* you can afford to wait before doing something heroic. So how do you determine whether breathing and circulation are present? Let's take each one separately.

Breathing and Circulation

Breathing: Sometimes (*if* you take those highly recommended few seconds) it is obvious that a person is still breathing even though he has "collapsed." It is obvious because you can see the chest moving or the mouth opening and closing with each breath; often a kind of snoring sound signals each breath. At other times, however, breathing can be more subtle, and you will have to "feel a breath" to make the determination—i.e., you will have to put your hand close to the mouth and/or nose to feel the air being exhaled with each breath.

Circulation: If the collapsed person has good color (pinkish, or healthy), you've got a good clue that circulation is intact. Actually, circulation involves two components—a pump (the heart) and something in the blood vessels (blood) to pump. The best way to tell whether the heart is working is to feel for a pulse, a procedure which requires that you know where to feel. There are several good locations to feel a pulse—including the one at the side of the wrist—but in an emergency the pulse in the neck (at the carotid artery) is often the easiest to feel. This pulse is best found by taking all four fingers (not your thumb) and placing them vertically in the groove on either side of the voicebox (adam's apple); usually the pulse is felt just below the level of the voicebox. (Practice on yourself right now so you can do it in an emergency.)

Again, if you can determine that breathing and circulation are intact, you can take time to make further decisions. And I stress that this is always worth doing, because most of the time you will have nothing further to do except make the person comfortable, raise the feet above chest level, loosen any clothing around the neck—and wait for him to wake up from what probably was a fainting spell. (At that point, of course, you will have to consider the need for further medical attention.) If, however, it becomes obvious that the person is not breathing and/or that circulation is absent (no pulse, the person is blue, etc.), then you must do something—namely, institute cardiopulmonary resuscitation.

Cardiopulmonary Resuscitation (CPR)

This is one of the great advances in the emergency care of the person whose life is immediately in danger, because it is a relatively safe and simple way of supporting breathing and circulation without any special equipment. The "cardio-" part of the procedure is sometimes referred to as external chest massage—i.e., a method of pushing on the outside of the chest in order to squeeze the heart between the front of the chest and the backbone, thereby forcing blood out of the heart and simulating its pumping function. The "-pulmonary" part refers to mouth-to-mouth breathing, which forces air into the lungs and thereby simulates breathing. Thus, the two done together in rhythmic fashion take over the two vital functions—breathing and circulation—until more definite help can be provided. Thousands of people today are alive who would have been dead without this procedure.

So far I have made this all sound simple. I must now confess that the proper performance of CPR requires practice under the instruction of someone skilled in the procedure. Consider taking advantage of the next opportunity that comes your way to learn CPR. There are very few investments which can pay you the dividend of saving a life. Many hospitals, companies, schools, medical societies, etc., offer periodic opportunities to learn this technique. The American Heart Association has taken special interest in the teaching of CPR, and you should check with the nearest local chapter about learning opportunities; the AHA has also published illustrated materials describing CPR which you can obtain from your local chapter or by writing the American Heart Association, 44 E. 23rd St., New York, N.Y. 10010.

I am convinced from personal experience that anyone who wants to can learn CPR. Most people will never have to use the procedure, but if the occasion arises it will be too late to learn.

Causes of Collapse

Having now discussed the basic approach to the situation of collapse, I can discuss more fully what actually causes a person to become suddenly unconscious. All tissues of the body need oxygen to live, but some are exquisitely sensitive to a lack of oxygen and will stop functioning (and die) very quickly in the absence of oxygen. The most sensitive tissues in terms of oxygen need are in the brain. Indeed, brain tissues cannot be deprived of oxygen for more than about four to six minutes without suffering permanent damage; even before that time, the parts of the brain that maintain consciousness will quit functioning properly, resulting in sudden unconsciousness—or what I am calling "collapse." This lack of oxygen to the brain can result from many situations, but the two most common causes are damage to the heart and interference with breathing. We can now list some of the specific problems in which collapse might occur and look at the unique factors in each:

1. *Heart attack:* A heart attack may or may not cause full collapse, depending on the effect on circulation. If the amount of heart muscle destroyed by a given heart attack is extensive enough and/or if the electrical system of the heart stops functioning, then circulation will cease and the individual will collapse; in such instances, CPR is necessary until more definitive treatment (electric shock, drugs, etc.) can be given by appropriately trained rescue squads or hospital personnel. However, many heart attack victims do not reach this state of full collapse initially; they may complain of severe pain and may experience great difficulty breathing, but they will be able to maintain enough circulation to allow for transport to the nearest appropriate medical facility. Obviously each case requires the kind of individual assessment described above.

2. *Choking:* Choking may cause collapse if blockage of the windpipe is enough to cut off the oxygen supply to the lungs and therefore to the brain. However, in the vast majority of choking situations, blockage is not complete,

and the situation can be corrected *if* the situation is not made worse by panicky reaction. One such reaction is blindly shoving fingers in the mouth to pull out whatever the person is choking on and instead pushing it down further in the throat. Another common error is pounding on the back with the person sitting upright; the result might be to loosen the object only to have it fall further down in the windpipe. The best approach to a person who appears to be choking is to attempt to calm that person down and determine if enough breathing is possible to transport the individual to a hospital where, with appropriate equipment and lighting and trained personnel, the obstructing material or object can be removed.

If, however, the person is truly "choking to death"— i.e., is turning blue and is unable to breath *or talk*—then something must be done immediately.

a. If the person involved is a small child, *first* turn the child upside down (hold him by the ankles, drape him over a leg, etc.) and slap sharply between the shoulder blades in an attempt to loosen the object or material. This approach may also be tried with an adult *if* it is possible to get the upper part of the body upside down.

b. With an appropriate device in the hands of someone trained to use it, it is possible to attempt to retrieve the blocking material. The most common setting for choking in an adult is while eating—particularly in an individual with false teeth who has been drinking and is consequently uncoordinated. Indeed, this kind of choking—on food— is so common and so often confused with a heart attack that it has been given the name "café coronary." (The major distinction between this and a massive heart attack is that the victim of choking will become very agitated but will not be able to breath *or speak;* the heart attack victim, if conscious, will be able to speak and breathe, though he may have difficulty doing so.) To attempt to better handle this common choking situation, an instrument—appropriately called ChokeSaver—has been devised by Dyna-Med, Incorporated, of Leucadia, California. The instrument consists of a curved plastic tweezer which can be inserted in the open position along the tongue to the back part of the throat with the handles remaining outside the mouth; when the handles are closed, the tweezer blades come together and the dull-edged teeth of the blades can grasp the meat or other food object to pull it out. Some states have introduced legislation to require all public eating places to have such a device. However, many physicians are concerned about the possible dangers of using this device without training—including the pushing of the food further down into the windpipe.

c. Another approach has recently been suggested by Dr. Henry Heimlich of the Jewish Hospital in Cincinnati; this approach is now appropriately called the "Heimlich maneuver." The basic idea is to suddenly, forcefully compress the abdomen in an attempt to force air out of the lungs and up the windpipe, thereby dislodging the choking material. The maneuver itself is nothing more than a super bear hug—encircling the person just above the belt line as he slumps forward and squeezing hard to force the diaphragm up, which compresses the lungs and forces air out. The same effect may be accomplished with a person on the floor or ground by rolling the victim on his back, placing one hand on top of the other in the upper abdomen while astride the victim, and pushing forcefully. This "Heimlich maneuver" has been reported widely, and, though Dr. Heimlich has tried it himself only in dog studies, he has received reports of successful saves from dozens of people. It has not been critically evaluated as yet.

d. I hesitate to mention a fourth approach because it

probably should be tried only by a trained and experienced person. On the other hand, in a desperate situation with death as the only alternative, anything can be justified. *Just between* the adam's apple and the smaller cartilage below it is a small indentation in the *center* of the neck. This indentation marks the location of a small membrane covering that part of the windpipe. Since this is below the voicebox and therefore below the point where most blocking objects (including food) get lodged, an opening into the windpipe at this point will usually provide a temporary passage for air. A small knife or other sharp object poked through this membrane may be sufficient to provide enough air passage to get the victim to a hospital; usually it is necessary to insert something small (like the barrel of a ballpoint pen with the insides removed) to keep the hole open. You can see why I hesitate to mention this, but I do so for completeness's sake. Permanent brain damage from choking can occur in minutes and in cases of dire emergency, there is no time to wait for trained rescuers.

3. *Massive bleeding:* The problem in this situation is that massive loss of blood means there is not enough fluid in the blood vessels to carry oxygen even if the heart is all right and breathing is occurring. And in this situation it does little good to support breathing and circulation with CPR unless blood (or a temporary substitute fluid) can be given. So the idea is to *prevent* such massive blood loss.

There is only one thing you have to know about how to stop bleeding: *sustained pressure directly on the site of bleeding*. Forget about pressure points and tourniquets or anything else you may have learned. All that is required to stop visible bleeding—even from a large artery—is the application of direct pressure *right on* the place of bleeding. If you have something sterile to use, fine. But the cleanest material available will do—sheets, towels, clothing articles, etc. Internal bleeding (bleeding that may be occurring inside the body but which you can't see) cannot be controlled in this fashion. And a large area of oozing-type bleeding is more difficult to control. But, in the vast majority of cases, bleeding can be controlled in the manner I have described, and that's all you need to know.

There are several ways of maintaining pressure sufficiently long to stop bleeding. The best way is to keep the pressure on with your own hands; that way you know what is happening. But, if you are alone and there are other areas of bleeding or other matters to attend to, you can wrap a belt or piece of cloth around and over the material pressed on the point of bleeding. A little ingenuity may be required but remember: *Direct pressure is the answer to bleeding.*

4. *Electrical injury:* The immediate cause of death in an electrical injury (lightning, hot wire, etc.) is stoppage of the heart due to interference with the electrical conducting system of the heart. CPR instituted soon enough may be life-saving since it may be sufficient to get the heart going again. However, treatment is complicated by the hazards of handling, for example, the victim in an auto accident with a hot wire draped over the car, etc. It is beyond the scope of this book to deal with such complicated rescue situations. But, if the victim is clear of any electrical hazard (such as when struck by lightning), immediate CPR is the answer. Later burn injuries may pose problems but the immediate situation requires restoration of breathing and heart action.

5. *Near-drowning:* Like electrical injuries, water im-
mersion can present somewhat complicated situations. But
the immediate problem is interference with breathing
which results in loss of consciousness and cardiac arrest.
And the immediate treatment of a victim of near-drowning
who may have a chance of survival is CPR—support of
breathing and circulation until treatment can be given
in a hospital.

6. *Massive blood clots to the lung (pulmonary emboli):*
Such clots interfere with blood circulation through the
lungs and therefore interfere with oxygen getting to the
body tissues. The sudden collapse of a victim of a *large*
lung blood clot is similar to that of a victim of a massive
heart attack; it is often difficult to tell the difference. But
the emergency treatment is the same for both—CPR.

7. *Stroke:* This term is applied to "cerebrovascular
accidents," that is, various causes of interference with
circulation to the brain. (The person may have a good
heart and a good breathing system, but, if blood can't get
to brain tissues, the effect will be the same as the situations
we have been discussing.) Most strokes do not result in
complete collapse; instead the victim will demonstrate
more localized problems—loss of speech, difficulty moving
extremities, etc. But, in a massive stroke with a large part
of the brain damaged, the result may be the same as in a
massive heart attack—sudden collapse. And since the
untrained person can't tell the difference and since the
basic needs are the same—namely support of breathing
and circulation—the answer is once again CPR until
further expertise is available. (See page 357.)

8. *Seizures:* These are one of the more common causes of collapse. (See page 340.) Generally it will be obvious that a person is having a seizure and that breathing and circulation are intact. Therefore, the situation can be handled much like a fainting spell—next on our list.

9. *Syncope* (fainting): The simple faint is the most common cause of a lapse of consciousness. It is embarrassing to start CPR on someone only to have him wake up quickly and demand to know what is going on. (But it is better for you to be embarrassed than for the patient to be dead—so, if you're not sure, start CPR.) Fainting is caused when the blood supply to the brain is reduced enough to cause loss of consciousness; the consequent falling to the ground is actually protective (unless the victim injures himself in the fall), since this will generally increase blood flow to the brain enough to awaken the sufferer. Indeed, you should be in no hurry to raise the person to a sitting position. All you need to do is make the person comfortable, raise the legs (which also promotes more blood to the brain), and loosen any tight clothing around the neck. Anyone who has fainted without obvious reason (such as sudden fright) should be seen by a doctor.

10. *Shock:* I mention this word only because it comes up so often in a discussion of life-threatening emergencies. (In some parts of the country the word "shock" is used to describe what is more commonly called a "stroke"— an episode wherein circulation to the brain is disturbed as described earlier.) A simple definition of shock is any condition in which the tissues of the body do not get

enough blood. By this definition, there are many possible causes of shock and most of the conditions I am speaking of in this section on life-threatening emergencies can lead to shock as I have just defined it. (As used more precisely in medicine, the word shock describes several complex situations which are beyond the scope of this book.) The point is that shock is something for doctors and the hospital to treat. Your job is to prevent it from developing —by the measures I have mentioned.

By now you should have the basic idea. Most life-threatening emergencies involve problems with breathing and circulation. It is sometimes difficult to tell which problem came first—the lack of oxygen or the lack of circulation. But in the immediate situation that question is academic. What the collapsed individual needs is CPR— support of breathing and circulation until further expertise is available. I hope I've convinced you to learn the technique at the earliest opportunity.

Head Injuries

Serious head injuries are usually obvious: the patient is unconscious, blood may be seen on the head or in the facial region, breathing may be abnormal, etc. Much more common—and diagnostically more troublesome—are the less obvious but potentially serious head injuries so common to the average household with children (falls from trees or highchairs, collisions on bikes and scooters, etc.). It is this kind of injury—which poses the question of whether to see the doctor or go to the hospital—that I will discuss. What applies to children in such cases, by the way, applies equally to adults.

If the child is found unconscious or becomes unconscious it is obvious that medical attention is necessary. One always faces the dilemma of whether it is safe to move a person who is unconscious, since there may be an associated neck fracture (or other injuries) which would make movement dangerous. If a child is found unconscious but is breathing normally, it is probably best—other circumstances allowing—to call for expert rescue squad assistance in moving the child. (If the child is awake, one should take a moment to see if he or she can move both arms and both legs; if not, again, it would be wise to call for expert assistance.)

Fortunately, the more common situation is for the child to be found crying (often hysterically) and frightened, but otherwise apparently all right. If it can be established that the child did not lose consciousness *and* if the victim can remember what happened, it is safe to keep the child at home under careful observation. Careful observation means observing the level of consciousness for the next twenty-four to forty-eight hours; it is *extremely* rare for a serious head injury not to "show itself" within this time period. Now we come to another problem—namely, the fact that it is normal for a child to become sleepy after any kind of prolonged excitement including getting hurt and having everybody fuss over him or her. Nor is it unusual for a child to get a headache and become nauseated after such an experience. And, as every mother knows, drowsiness, headaches, and vomiting are signs of serious head injury. Well, they can be, but usually they are not. And that's the problem—how is a mother to know?

Quite frankly, there are no easy guidelines to what constitutes serious drowsiness or headaches or vomiting. Generally, drowsiness from which the child cannot be easily aroused, headaches which are not relieved by the appropriate amount of aspirin (and some rest), or vomiting which is projectile (shooting out) and occurs later are the things to worry about. But I fully appreciate the anxiety felt by a parent whose child is experiencing any kind of problem after a head injury and I see no reason why such a child shouldn't be checked out if only for "peace of mind"—so call your doctor or go to the emergency room.

When you do go for medical evaluation you will be asked about the loss of consciousness and the child will be questioned for memory of the event. In the absence of obvious signs of serious head injury (unequal pupil size, blood or other fluid from the ears, abnormal neurological signs, etc.), these are the best clues as to the seriousness of the injury. The doctor will usually look in the back of the eyes with an ophthalmoscope, though this may be difficult in a small child who hasn't yet been impressed with the value in life of occasionally holding still. The doctor should also look in the ears and check out a few reflexes.

Now we come to the question of whether or not to order a skull X ray. It is often done for possible legal reasons. I say this because it has been well demonstrated that in the absence of clinical evidence of a serious head injury (what the patient demonstrates), the skull X rays will invariably show nothing of significance. And it is often frightening for a small child to have skull X rays—strapped in, kept motionless, and a big machine pointed at him. But parents are worried, doctors "don't want to take any chances," and so skull X rays are often ordered. But, if a doctor tries to explain why he doesn't think they are necessary and if he is willing to say that he wouldn't get any for his child under the same circumstances, you are probably getting very good advice.

Generally, if a child has suffered definite loss of consciousness and/or cannot remember what happened, the doctor will want to hospitalize the child for twenty-four hour observation. Occasionally under these circumstances, if the doctor can be convinced that home observation will be just as reliable as hospital nursing observation, he will allow the child to go home. Whatever the decision, any child should be observed as described above during the first twenty-four to forty-eight hours after a head injury. Observation for level of consciousness should mean arousing the child (if sleeping) every one to two hours; "arousing" doesn't mean that the child has to get up and exercise, but it does mean that it should be reasonably easy to awaken the child enough so he wants to know what all the fuss is about.

Sometimes after even a mild head injury, an individual will experience what is described as a "posttraumatic syndrome"—meaning a collection of symptoms that occurs after a head injury but for which no obvious cause can be found. These symptoms include persistent headaches, tiring easily, memory defects, difficulty concentrating, etc. Occasionally these symptoms last six months before improving, though usually they disappear before that with appropriate medications and reassurance.

Any primary care physician (including emergency-room physicians) should be capable of evaluating head injuries. If there is any evidence of a serious problem, the neurosurgeon will be consulted. While skull X rays and other more sophisticated tests such as Echo and EEG studies may be useful, in any serious problem case the neurosurgeon will probably want to resort to cerebral angiography for definitive diagnosis. This is a procedure where dye is injected into the vessels leading to the brain and X rays are taken outlining the brain blood vessels, thereby demonstrating where bleeding might be occurring. Recently a new technique called CAT (Computerized Axial Tomography) has been developed which allows similar diagnosis without the dangers of injecting dye into the brain circulation; however, the machines used for CAT are very expensive and not yet generally available. As they become available, they will make diagnosis of some brain injuries (and other brain problems) easier and safer than using angiography.

Poisoning

Consistent with the purpose of this book, there are four things everyone should know about poisoning:

1. *Prevention:* Most poisoning incidents could have been prevented with thought and foresight. I often recommend that a parent literally get down on hands and knees and "walk" around the entire house (and garage and yard) and from that vantage point see what a child sees and might get into. (You risk your family and neighbors wondering whether they should get you fitted for a straitjacket, but it's worth the gamble.)

2. *Phone:* One of the first things you should do when you move into new living quarters is to get the phone number of the nearest Poison Information Center and post that number prominently by your phone. This number can be obtained from the medical society or from the phone company.

3. *Vomiting:* Every home should have a bottle of *syrup of ipecac,* which can be bought without prescription at any drugstore (many drugstores give it for nothing). Ipecac will induce vomiting, which is the initial treat-

ment in the majority of ingested poisonings. *You should never give ipecac (or anything else) until you have called the Poison Information Center for advice.* Some substances (lyes, corrosives, petroleum products, etc.) should not be treated by inducing vomiting. But many ingestions are so treated initially, and with ipecac on hand you can get an important head start.

4. *Surface "poisoning"*: The treatment of any potential poison which spills onto the body (or into the eyes or mouth or nose or ears, etc.) is *immediate and thorough rinsing with water.* Rinse with the most water as fast as you can—hoses, showers, buckets, faucets, etc. If clothing is involved, get it off while rinsing. Don't use anything but plain old water. Rinse with water even before you call for further advice. Seconds may count in the outcome. If the eyes are involved, have someone hold open the lids while water is flushed into them for at least 20 minutes. (See page 290.)
That's really all you need to know about poisoning.

Burns

Two areas of burn treatment deserve mention in this book: the immediate treatment and the possibilities for long-term treatment of severe burns. First, the immediate treatment of burns can be summarized by saying "the less the better." Which is an oversimplified warning against putting butter, creams, grease, etc., on burns as first-aid treatment. Now let's be more specific.

There are three major determinants of the severity of a burn—the *degree* of burn, the *amount* (area) involved, and the *location* of a burn. Let's discuss each of these factors:

1. *Degree:* First degree means redness without blistering (like a minor sunburn.) Second means redness *with* blistering. And third means destruction of the full layer of skin and often of deeper structures; third-degree burns are usually whitish in color and without sensation. It often takes twenty-four to forty-eight hours before a final decision can be made about burns that are initially between the second and third degrees; this decision becomes important in terms of treatment.

   Minor first-degree burns can be handled at home. Submerging the affected area in cold water (or wrapping it with wet bandages) immediately after the burn for about thirty minutes will reduce pain and damage. Usually the burned area will change colors and heal within several weeks. If the area becomes increasingly tender and pussy, suggesting infection, medical attention must be sought. Leaving the burned area open to air and keeping it clean is the best treatment after the cold application.

   Small areas of second-degree burns can be handled initially the same way—cold water. Then, when blister formation has stopped, the blisters may be punctured (using sterile technique), leaving the skin in place; the area is then wrapped with sterile dressings (often coated with petrolatum or similar material). Dressings can be changed periodically and healing usually is accomplished within two to three weeks. This kind of burn usually requires the attention of someone capable of doing what has just been described. If the area is very small, it can probably be handled at home by keeping the area clean and letting nature take its course. The blisters will break by themselves.

Third-degree burns *always* need medical attention. Skin grafting may be required, and that decision must be made by a competent physician with appropriate experience. As mentioned before, it is not always possible to tell initially whether a burn will turn out to be second or third degree and examination twenty-four to forty-eight hours later may be required.

2. *Amount:* The larger the area of second- and third-degree burns, the more serious. This is partially due to increased fluid loss and possibility for infection. Any extensive burn should be wrapped in clean cloth and seen immediately at the nearest appropriate medical facility.

3. *Location:* Burns of the face, hands, joint areas, and genitalia are always potentially more dangerous because of possible cosmetic and functional damage. Any burn of these areas except very minor first-degree ones should be evaluated by an appropriate physician. Also of concern is inhalation of hot gases or flames; this should be suspected in any burn of the head and neck area. Such inhalation burns can result in serious breathing system damage.

We come now to the question of where to go for more than minor burn problems. The very initial treatment of serious burns is somewhat standard—administration of intravenous fluids, control of pain, and so on. As soon as possible, however, such burn cases should be transferred to the nearest facility specializing in burn treatment. Burn therapy today has become very specialized and sophisticated and requires intensive care and modern knowledge; only a few hospitals are capable of meeting this challenge. Fortunately most hospitals recognize their limitations and are only too happy to transfer patients with severe burns. The doctors most involved with burn care are general and plastic surgeons. Aggressive skin grafting (within days) has improved survival and function dramatically. This is one area of medicine where expertise is limited and worth traveling to get.

Joint Injuries

The "sprain" injury is one of the most common "emergencies" of life. I put emergency in quotes because while it is not a life-and-death emergency, a sprain of a key joint may be potentially very serious.

For purposes of this book, the most important discussion is the proper way to handle joint injuries at the time they occur. And the single most important point to be made is this: Avoid *all* weight bearing on the injured joint until it can be determined whether serious damage has occurred. If this rule is carefully followed, there is no reason to rush to the hospital or doctor's office with a sprain injury. But this means that the weekend basketball player with a sprain must stop playing, that the tennis buff must not finish the match.

In addition to stopping all weight bearing, *elevation* (above chest level) of the injured joint plus an *ice-cold pack* (any reasonable way of getting cold on the joint will do) for twenty-four hours are helpful. If at the end of twenty-four hours of such rest the joint is still painful or swollen, then it *is* appropriate to visit a doctor or hospital. At this point, a visit directly to an orthopedic surgeon will save time and money since that is the doctor to whom a primary care physician will refer you for any serious joint injury.

The following kinds of joint injury deserve to be shown to a physician immediately—before the twenty-four-hour waiting period described above:

1. Any obviously severe injury—marked by gross deformity of the joint, severe pain, severe swelling, etc. A certain amount of individual judgment is required, but, if there is a chance that the sprain is serious, see a doctor.

2. Any injury to the knee joint should be taken seriously, since this joint is crucial and since any weight put on it could cause further damage. The same could be said for any other joint, of course, but I find that people often take the knee joint less seriously than they should.

A quick word about X-ray studies. Routine X rays demonstrate bone injuries and do not routinely show injuries to the ligaments and cartilages—which are the joint structures that get injured in a sprain. Routine X rays are certainly worth taking to rule out unsuspected fractures—particularly so-called avulsion fractures, in which a piece of bone is "pulled off" due to the severity of the sprain. When it is important to demonstrate more clearly the soft tissue structures of joints (ligaments and cartilages), then xerography—a special X-ray technique which more clearly demonstrates such structures—and/or arthrography—where dye is injected into the joint to outline these soft tissue structures—may be employed. Arthrography is being used increasingly to clarify joint injuries which do not improve with the conservative care of rest and elevation.

Sometimes a sprained joint is put in a cast even though there is no fracture involved. Such treatment allows the joint to recuperate without weight bearing or other stress and will allow the person to be more mobile than might otherwise be possible.

There are several controversies in the management of severe joint injuries. Usually they involve the question of whether immediate surgery or more conservative treatment is best. There are no easy answers to some of these questions and the good judgment of an experienced orthopedic surgeon is the best I can suggest. Finding such a physician in the middle of emergency circumstances (like a ski slope) can be difficult; you should not feel embarrassed to request transfer from such a circumstance to your home hospital where you have an orthopedic surgeon you know and trust. As pointed out initially, as long as you keep weight off the joint there is little further damage you can do.

Lacerations (*Cuts*)

The question usually is this: Does Sally's cut or Tommy's gash (or your own) need to be sutured? There is no simple answer; when there is a question, the judgment of experience is usually necessary to decide. The factors that a physician will take into consideration in making the decision include the following:

1. *The location of the cut:* If the cut is located where appearance is important (face, bikini territory), suturing may be done for cosmetic reasons. If the cut is located over a joint or other area of movement, sutures may be necessary lest the cut constantly open and delay healing. *Any* cut of the lip involving the border between lip and skin should be evaluated; the same is true of any cut of the eyelid involving the margin of the lid.

2. *The age of the patient:* Small kids have a well-honed and God-given talent for pulling apart any bandage devised by man. Therefore, cuts that might be handled with taping or butterflies in an older child or adult might be sutured in a smaller child just to increase the chances of keeping the wound edges together for the required healing time. (Actually, kids can do a pretty good job on stitches too, but it takes more effort.)

3. *The nature of the wound:* If the cut edges are under tension and pulling apart, sutures are more necessary than if the edges fall nicely together without tension.

The name of the game is to cover open wounds with skin—which speeds healing and minimizes the chance of infection. Usually this can be accomplished by pulling the skin edges together; sometimes a skin graft from elsewhere on the patient's body becomes necessary. If a chunk of tissue (or a body part) is cut off it is worth bringing it in to the doctor—it may be usable in the grafting process.

Healing depends on several factors, including:

1. *Age and general medical condition of the patient:* Generally, the elderly patient or the patient with other complicating medical problems (particularly diabetes) heals more slowly.

2. *Location of the cut:* Certain areas of the body (such as the lower part of the leg) have a poor blood supply and therefore will not heal as quickly. Also, as suggested above, cuts over movable parts of the body (such as joints) will heal more slowly unless that part is immobilized in a splint or heavy bandage.

3. *Wound care:* Keeping the wound clean and dry will promote healing, as will elevating the injured part

of the body when possible. Injured tissues need rest for healing, and any way this can be accomplished will be helpful.

Once the determination has been made that sutures are necessary, the question of "what kind of doctor should do it" arises. It is impossible to generalize in answer to this question. Small cuts in areas not critical to appearance can be sutured by almost anyone with reasonably good results. Larger, more irregular cuts in areas of cosmetic concern require some skill and experience. The only recommendation I can honestly offer is this: Ask the physician with whom you are dealing if he is capable of "handling" the latter type of cut. Such a question will put him on notice that you are concerned, but it will not rule out his doing the necessary repair if he feels qualified. (Obviously the way in which you ask the question will have much to do with the kind of response you will get. A suggested way: "Is this something you can do, doctor, or do you think someone else is required?") Many general physicians and pediatricians have had considerable experience and have developed excellent skills in wound repairs; for routine cuts, they can be every bit as good as general or plastic surgeons.

Finally, a reminder that a cut must be sutured as soon as possible. Most physicians will refuse to suture a wound more than six to eight hours old because by that time the open area is contaminated with bacteria and if the wound is closed over by sutures there is a good chance that infection under the sutured edges will occur. Such a wound must be left open to heal—which takes much longer and leaves a greater scar. When in doubt, then, check it out as soon as possible.

Since recommendations concerning tetanus boosters

have recently changed, and since tetanus immunity is confusing, *and* since several hundred needless deaths still occur every year from tetanus—the subject deserves comment.

Tetanus is a disease which results from a poison released by a germ (*Clostridium tetani*) which can grow only in the absence of oxygen. Tetanus germs are everywhere and ready to crawl into even the slightest cut. (Deep puncture-type wounds are the most susceptible, but any kind of wound is potentially a home for these germs.) The only sure protection, therefore, is immunization.

There are two basic kinds of immunization—active, where the body is stimulated to produce its own antibodies, and passive, where antibodies developed elsewhere are put into your body for short-term coverage. Active immunization is achieved by, first, a basic series of shots, several months apart, followed by a booster about a year later. In kids, the tetanus shot is part of the DPT shot— the T stands for tetanus, the D for diphtheria and the P for pertussis (whooping cough); these are given three times during the first year. In an adult who escaped such basic immunization as a child, three shots four to eight weeks apart followed by a booster a year later are required.

Once basic immunization (the series of shots just described) is achieved, a booster shot is required periodically to keep the immunized state active. In kids, after the basic series, this is accomplished according to the regular immunization schedule, as outlined in the section on immunizations (page 315). In adults, routine boosters (in the absence of cuts and injuries) are recommended every seven to ten years.

If an injury, puncture wound, or cut occurs, a booster should be given if more than five years have elapsed since the last booster. (Also important is proper cleaning of the

wound; soap and water are sufficient for minor wounds.)
If no basic immunization has ever been given—and this
is not uncommon in older people—then both kinds of
immunization (as described above) must be given: (1). A
shot of tetanus immune globulin (containing human antibodies) is first given to cover the situation until active
immunization can be developed. It is this shot—which
used to be obtained from horses—that is associated with
bad memories about "reactions" to tetanus shots. The
shots used today are prepared from humans and may give
occasionally severe local reactions but only *very* rarely
the more serious generalized reactions. (2). At the same
time, a program of basic immunization as outlined above
(three shots) is started with the first of the three required
shots. Arrangements must be made to receive two more
shots during the next several months.

In other words, authorities now suggest that a booster
every year is not required and in fact may be harmful.
The most important way of getting the right number of
shots is to *keep your own record:* hospital and office
records are not available when you need them. Every time
you get a tetanus shot, have the person giving it write
down the date and kind of shot and keep that record
in your wallet.

Nosebleed (*Epistaxis*)

Ninety-five percent of nosebleeds occur in the anterior
(front) portion of the nose and are therefore usually easily
controlled; the other five percent occur in the posterior
(back) part of the nose (obviously) and usually require the
insertion of a "posterior pack"—which requires the
special skills of a physician. The vast majority of anterior
nosebleeds can be controlled at home (or wherever they

occur), thereby avoiding the cost and inconvenience of a trip to the hospital or doctor. Such control is achieved as follows:

1. Lean forward (to avoid swallowing blood, which is unpleasant and may cause vomiting). Do so in front of a clock.

2. You should now be asking: Why the clock? (If you did not question that advice, I have some good stock in the Brooklyn Bridge I would like to speak to you about.) The clock is to assure that you apply pressure to the anterior part of your nose by pinching the nostrils for a full 15 minutes *by the clock* (or your wristwatch, if you can see it while pinching).

3. The pinching is done by closing your nostrils firmly with your thumb and index finger. If you do it properly, those fingers will get tired, and you will need to relieve them with the same fingers of the opposite hand. But remember: Do not release pressure until fifteen minutes have passed *by the clock.* If, after the above, bleeding continues or recurs, pinch your nose again and head for the nearest doctor or hospital.

If nosebleeds become recurrent or severe, obviously you must seek medical attention. If you have any suspicion that nosebleeds are related to other medical problems, such as hypertension, you should also seek attention. But most nosebleeds are related to blows to the nose, dried nasal linings from low humidity, or the "finger in the nose."

After a nosebleed (however treated), lying down while avoiding hot foods, smoking, and vigorous blowing will help minimize a recurrence. If a nasal pack is inserted, be sure to obtain careful direction as to its care and the time of removal; the pack is not to be left in until it rots away.

Rib Injury

Few people make it through life without receiving an injury to the chest wall—whether it be a slip on the ice or a Saturday night elbow in the ribs. And, either immediately or within a few hours, localized pain follows—made worse by deep breathing or movement or touching. The next day it's worse, so a trip to the hospital or doctor's office is made. And the usual pattern is to X ray the ribs; ninety percent of the time the report is negative for fracture. The facts of the matter are these:

1. Injury to the ribs is very painful, whether it is "simply" a bruise or a fracture.

2. The pain of such an injury lasts for two to four weeks —so be prepared.

3. Unless the rib injury was associated with a blow of severe force (such as in an auto accident), there is little danger of associated injury to underlying lung, spleen, or liver tissue. The ribs are encased in a solid sheath of muscle which keeps them in place, even when cracked.

In light of the above, my own practice is as follows:

1. If the lungs sound normal, I seldom take X rays— unless there are legal or clear medical reasons to do so. Since the pain of bruise and fracture is about the same, and since they both last for about the same time, the distinction is academic. In other words, why take X rays if it isn't going to change the treatment?

2. I seldom use rib binders. The idea behind the rib binder is to wrap it on tight enough to decrease movement of the rib cage—which therefore cuts down on the pain. But cutting down that much on chest wall

movement also increases the risk of developing pneumonia, especially in older people. So I usually just tell the sad story of the two to four weeks ahead and prescribe some pain medicine for use (especially at night when pain from rolling around in bed causes fitful sleep). In cases of severe pain, injection of anesthesia into the appropriate area may be useful.

The truth of the matter is that, no matter what is done, you'll get better if it's just a simple rib blow. Knowing that, you may want to stay home and save your money. Obviously, if the pain is accompanied by other significant symptoms—coughing, bloody sputum, fever, etc.—you should see a doctor.

Heatstroke

True heatstroke is very rare, but it presents a real emergency when it does occur. The hallmarks of true heatstroke are a rather sudden loss of consciousness accompanied by very high fever *and no sweating*. In this combination of circumstances, the victim should be covered with cold packs and transported immediately to the nearest medical facility. Much more common than true heatstroke are conditions described as heat exhaustion or heat prostration. In these cases there may be loss of consciousness or a feeling of fainting—and there is also *profuse sweating*. Usually movement to a cool place and elevation of the legs is sufficient immediate treatment. Since the underlying problem is usually salt and/or water depletion, these must be replaced. Since all "heat illnesses" may be related to underlying medical problems, they should be reported to the victim's source of medical care.

Frostbite

The keynote is prevention: "Keep warm, keep moving, keep dry." Frostbites, like burns, are described in degrees —first degree being without blistering or peeling, second with blistering and peeling, and third being actual skin death. Early warning signs of impending frostbite include numbness, prickling, and itching; that's the time to take action. The immediate treatment recommendations from the experts change almost every year. The value of rapid rewarming is still a matter of controversy. What seems clear is that rubbing or exercising frozen tissues in case of third-degree frostbite causes further destruction; obviously, this should *not* be done. Medical advice is imperative for third-degree frostbite.

2

Heart Disease

For most people, "heart disease" is synonymous with "heart attack." There are, however, many other kinds of heart disease besides the disease process which leads to a heart attack. It is beyond the scope of this book to discuss all heart disease, but the following heart problems are discussed separately in this section:

- Coronary artery disease
- Palpitations (irregular or pounding heartbeats)
- Rheumatic fever (a disease in which the heart is a major concern)
- Heart failure
- Heart murmur

The heart is composed of three major functional parts: an electrical system which directs and coordinates the proper beating of the heart, four chambers composed of muscle which respond to the electrical system by contracting, and four valves which direct the flow of blood through the heart as it beats. All of these parts are supplied with blood (needed by the heart just like every other part of the body) from the coronary arteries—two arteries which form smaller branches that eventually supply all parts of the heart. Finally, the heart is surrounded by a sac called the pericardium which forms a protective environment within which the heart can do its work. I have listed these parts to remind you that "heart disease" can mean trouble with any or all of these components. The most common form of heart disease is the process of atherosclerosis (so-called "hardening of the arteries") as it affects the coronary arteries which supply blood to the heart. It is this disease process which leads to "heart attacks," and it is this disease which is appropriately described as our nation's "No. 1 killer." Therefore, I have devoted a large section to the prevention, diagnosis, and treatment of this disease under the title "Coronary Artery Disease."

One form of heart disease deserves a quick mention— so-called "congenital heart disease," a phrase which refers to disease present at birth. Usually the problems associated with congenital heart disease become obvious early in life (or even at the time of birth) and become the province of the pediatrician and pediatric heart specialists. Occasionally, a heart problem present since birth does not cause trouble until somewhat later in life. One special problem is the "heart murmur" in childhood; since this is so common, it is discussed separately under "Heart Murmurs."

A word on "heart specialists" is in order. As pointed out in Part I, any doctor can describe himself in any manner he wishes. In the field of heart disease, many older physicians have become known as "heart specialists" by virtue of long experience and consequent competence in diagnosing and treating heart disease. The younger physician follows a more formal path of training and experience to the point where he can be legitimately described as a "heart specialist." That training involves a standard program in internal medicine (three years after graduation from medical school), followed by special training at the fellowship level in heart disease. Following fellowship training in heart disease, most doctors will go into the practice of general internal medicine with a special emphasis on heart disease that will lead in later years to exclusive practice as a cardiologist; other doctors will go immediately into the exclusive practice of cardiology. All of this is somewhat academic since no modern cardiologist can practice effectively apart from a well-equipped hospital which will exert some control over the quality of its staff. The questions usually arise when a person is being treated by a general practitioner for an instance of heart disease that might merit more intensive investigation and different treatment. There are no easy rules; as with any health problem, if satisfaction is not obtained after a patient expresses concern to a doctor, the patient should not hesitate to seek a different opinion—in this case from a recognized cardiologist. Such a doctor is recognized by the kind of training described above; usually local or state medical societies can suggest nearby specialists, but this is another instance in which accurate "inside" information is most useful.

Finally, as part of this introductory statement on heart disease, a word about chest pain is in order. Without question, this is one of the most difficult symptoms to interpret for both lay people and physicians. First, pain in the chest —like pain in the abdomen—can have many significant causes. Second, most chest pain is *not* serious. But, third, serious chest pain may not *seem* serious; we all know people with heart attacks who took too long to get to a doctor or hospital because of what they thought was an "upset stomach." All of this adds up to the adage: When in doubt, check it out.

The chest (or thorax) contains three important structures—all of which are sources of trouble. As described earlier, the *heart* can cause pain for many different reasons; most fearsome, however, is the pain caused by so-called "heart attacks." The *lungs,* contained in linings called the pleura, can also cause pain for many different reasons, including pleurisy, pneumonia, an embolus (blood clot) in the lung, etc. The *esophagus* (the food pipe leading from the throat to the stomach) is less likely to be the source of chest pain but must always be thought of as a possibility.

In addition to these major structures are the muscles, nerves, ribs and cartilages that make up the chest wall or "rib cage." In fact, most chest pains are due to usually minor but often irritating afflictions of these chest wall structures—such as viral infections of the cartilages in the rib cage or muscle strain of the muscles between the ribs (the intercostal muscles). Fortunately, these pains can usually be recognized as not being due to more serious problems.

Chest pains which are *fleeting* (seconds in duration), *variable* in location (in back one time and in front another), associated with movement or change in *position* and *not* associated with fever, difficulty in breathing, or marked sweating—these chest pains are usually not serious. One can afford to wait a day or two if they occur only occasionally before seeking medical help.

The following kinds of chest pain, however, must be investigated immediately:

1. Any chest pain associated with marked sweating, difficulty in breathing, or fever above 101° (orally).

2. Any chest pain which increases in frequency, intensity, or persistency.

3. Any chest pain in someone with a previous history of chest-located disease—such as a previous heart attack or blood clot in the lung.

4. Any chest pain marked by nagging persistency—that is, constant, annoying, and not relieved by change in position or change of mental occupation. In other words, a chest pain that causes you to lie down for a half hour instead of watching your favorite TV program, or awakens you from good sleep and persists, should be checked.

And, again, since pain in the chest may be life-threatening, it should be investigated more readily than other kinds of pain.

Coronary Artery Disease (*Heart Attacks*)

This is such a serious disease, and one affecting so many people, that it is useful to have a basic understanding of the disease process—so that's where we'll start.

The Process

The basic disease underlying coronary artery disease is atherosclerosis—a fancy word describing a poorly understood process by which fatlike material is deposited in the inner lining of blood vessels eventually leading to their blockage. (The term arteriosclerosis is also often used, and sometimes the phrase "hardening of the arteries" is used to describe the process we are talking about. It is not accurate, but does convey the fact that there is a problem with blood vessels resulting in a compromise of blood flow.) Ultimately the answer to coronary artery disease lies in a better understanding of the process of atherosclerosis and a consequent ability to prevent it from occurring. Until that point of medical knowledge is reached, we are left with "second-best" measures—minimizing known risk factors and emphasizing early diagnosis and treatment.

Atherosclerosis can affect many blood vessels, but we are now concerned with describing what happens when it occurs in the coronary arteries—the two arteries which direct blood as it is pumped out of the heart and back to the heart. In other words, the heart, which pumps blood to all parts of the body, must get its own blood supply through vessels just like all other organs; it cannot absorb necessary oxygen and nutrients directly from the blood inside its chambers. As these arteries and their branches become plugged, blood flow to the heart is diminished and the heart is deprived of the oxygen and nutrients necessary for the heart muscle to function. In the earlier stages of this "plugging," the heart muscle reacts to its diminished blood supply by sending out warning signals of pain—so-called "angina." At this point, the heart muscle is in trouble but not yet down for the count. As the process of plugging continues *or* when the work of the heart is increased (as may occur when the victim is shoveling snow, for example), a point will be reached where oxygen demand is greater than supply and the affected area of heart muscle "dies"—that is, it is irreversibly damaged. *When actual tissue death has occurred* we describe the event as a myocardial infarction (MI) or "heart attack."

I have described these developing stages of ischemia (poor blood supply) so that you clearly understand that a "heart attack" is the final step in a long process of decreased blood flow to the heart muscle. The obvious concern is to slow or prevent the plugging and diagnose and treat the victim before an actual heart attack occurs. I have described this process of plugging as a long one; some experts say it begins the day we are born. That may be overly dramatic, but autopsies done on young soldiers indicate that even in our teens the process is well underway. I have also described a sequence of events that may not always occur. For example, the first warning of trouble may be heart failure or disturbance of heart rhythm or even sudden death—all without any warning chest pain; this is part of what makes coronary artery disease so frightening. But in most cases there are warning signs.

Symptoms

I have described above the classical "cry for help" of the ischemic heart as angina—chest pain. Angina is often subtle and described best in terms other than pain: as a sensation of squeezing, burning, pressing, choking, aching, or, classically, as "an elephant sitting on my chest." It is often discounted as "heartburn." It may also, however, be sudden and excruciating pain.

There are other characteristics of angina which may be useful in distinguishing it from other causes of distress. Distribution of distress, relationship to exercise, response to rest, response to nitroglycerin medication—all are useful but not definitive in diagnosis.

Indeed, the most important point I can make in this section is that there is no certain way to diagnose coronary artery disease by its symptoms. And, if the doctor has trouble deciding on the basis of symptoms, you should be even more careful to have suspicious symptoms checked by your doctor or the nearest emergency room.

Diagnosis

Ideally, one would like to diagnose coronary artery disease before an actual heart attack occurs. As indicated in the previous section, symptoms are often less than clear-cut—and, even when the story is classical, the doctor will need tests to either confirm or rule out coronary artery disease. Certain tests are useful in deciding how advanced coronary artery disease may be and/or whether an actual heart attack has occurred.

First is the *ECG*. The electrocardiogram is still the mainstay of routine diagnosis. Useful as it is, it does not represent a final word. All too many cases of normal ECG's followed by proven coronary artery disease exist. Increasing use is now being made of the stress ECG—an ECG performed under various stress conditions, such as climbing stairs, riding a bike, or performing on a treadmill. The stress ECG is particularly useful in cases where coronary artery disease is strongly suspected but the routine ECG shows nothing.

Second are *blood enzyme studies*. These are done routinely today in any suspected heart attack. They are very useful in questionable cases but cannot be taken alone as evidence of an actual attack.

Coronary angiography is a third test. It is a technique whereby dye is injected into the coronary arteries (under X-ray guidance) and motion pictures are taken of the dye as it passes through the coronary arterial circulation. This technique has revolutionized the diagnosis and treatment of coronary artery disease since it provides, for the first time, a direct look at the coronary arteries and their branches; guesswork based on secondary evidence from blood tests and ECG's is thereby eliminated. There are several reasons, however, why this procedure is not used on a routine basis. First, the cost in terms of equipment and personnel is enormous; the procedure must be done under conditions similar to the operating room with preparation for emergencies that can develop during the procedure. Second, even under the best of conditions, there are risks involved; done by experienced operators, risk of death is under one percent but there are other complications short of death that vary from one to seven percent. The obvious question is, Who should have this done? At least the following groups of people should be considered:

a. Patients in whom coronary artery disease is strongly suspected but in whom diagnosis has not been possible. I refer to those patients whose history is very suggestive of coronary artery disease but whose ECG's, even under stress conditions, have not made a definite diagnosis possible. Angiography can almost always provide the answer as to whether significant coronary artery disease exists.

b. Patients who have become "cardiac neurotics." In this age of continual warning about heart disease, some people develop incapacitating fear of coronary artery disease. On occasion, angiography is justified to demonstrate that no coronary artery disease exists.

c. Patients who are to be considered for coronary bypass surgery. Indeed, it is this technique which has made such surgery possible. Only by visualizing the coronary arteries can a decision be made as to whether surgery is feasible. (See pages 124–126.)

The ideal diagnostic technique would be one that combines the accuracy of angiography with the safety of the

ECG. As yet that is not available, but studies are continuing in this direction.

It should be obvious from the outline I have provided that diagnosis sometimes involves a great deal of skill and judgment. When heart disease is suspected, the skills of a cardiologist are very much in order. Usually a primary care physician will refer a patient when such skill is needed, but no one should hesitate to make a direct appointment with a cardiologist when concern is great.

Treatment

Again, the goal of treatment ideally would be to prevent a heart attack from occurring. Unfortunately, once coronary artery disease has occurred, there is no way to reverse or remove the existing fatty material, and attention therefore must be directed to preventing further damage (see pages 128–132) and treating the existing situation, both medically and socially.

Medical treatment of existing coronary artery disease involves careful attention to the complications of diminished circulation to the heart. These complications may include heart failure or problems with heart rhythm (arrhythmias), both of which can be helped enormously through careful treatment. Social treatment involves an assessment of life-style and rearrangement where possible of stresses which might contribute to a worsening of coronary artery disease or might add an unnecessary work load to an already damaged heart. However, care must always be taken not to unreasonably heighten anxiety, which may turn a productive person into a nervous wreck.

The single most important and controversial advance in treatment of coronary artery disease in recent years is the development of coronary artery bypass surgery (hereinafter referred to as bypass). The theory is simple and direct. A vein is taken from the leg and used to bypass the area of blockage (as identified via coronary angiography) thereby restoring better blood flow to the heart. Such surgery, which involves open heart and lung bypass techniques, is now almost routine in terms of the mechanics involved. But considerable controversy, mainly on two counts, surrounds this new surgical "miracle."

1. *Who should have the surgery?* Apart from the fact that there are not enough surgeons and facilities to perform surgery on everyone with coronary artery disease, there is increasing evidence that only certain kinds of patients with coronary artery disease will benefit. These indications are constantly being refined and changed. Factors which contribute to a decision as to whether surgery is feasible include the general health of the patient, the location of the coronary artery disease (which vessels are involved and the technical problems posed), the adequacy of medical (that is, nonsurgical) treatment, etc.

2. *Will the surgery last?* It has been well demonstrated that, in carefully selected cases, bypass can offer dramatic relief of anginal pain. However, there are two areas of postoperative developments for which final answers are not in yet:

   a. Will the grafted vein remain an open, efficient blood channel over a long period of time? We now know that about thirty percent of grafts will become clogged within a few years.

   b. There is also increasing evidence of an increased risk of heart attacks following bypass surgery. Since the surgery is designed to avoid such damage, this in part detracts from the value of the surgery. As of this writing it is difficult to evaluate the impact of this evidence but it bears watching.

In sum, then, bypass is a procedure now being widely used without the kind of knowledge we need to recommend it without reservation. Studies are underway to clarify the role of bypass in prolongation of life. Until better answers are in we must regard it as less than a surgical miracle and reserve it for situations that will clearly not benefit from further nonsurgical therapy.

Once a heart attack has occurred, there is much that can be done to prevent complications and minimize further damage. The following is a brief listing of some of the more important treatment possibilities available:

First are the *coronary care units.* It is now clear that the majority of heart attack victims suffer rhythm problems during the first twenty-four hours after an attack. These arrhythmias will often, without treatment, lead to death. This is why it is absolutely essential to seek treatment *immediately* when a heart attack is suspected; waiting even an hour may be fatal. Since the emphasis on monitoring heart attack victims in special units where nurses are in constant attendance, the mortality rate *in hospitals* from heart attacks has been halved. But that kind of salvage is possible *only* if the heart attack victim is brought to the hospital promptly.

Obviously it is important to know whether a given hospital has an appropriately equipped and staffed coronary care unit. In cases of known heart disease where the chance of a heart attack is more than routinely possible, this kind of knowledge should be obtained before an emergency arises. A frank discussion with your doctor or clinic is warranted. Ideally, hospitals should be clearly identified as to their capacity to handle heart attack victims. But, until that has been accomplished, potential users of coronary care units (and that really includes any adult) should find out before the fact.

Second is *temporary electrical pacing.* The use of electrical impulses to cause the heart to beat when damage to the heart's own electrical system has occurred represents an exciting development in the care of heart attack victims. We are now much more aware of those heart attacks which are likely to cause damage that will result in stoppage of the heart. In these instances, a temporary wire is inserted into the heart through a vein leading to it, and electrical impulses are supplied to the heart when and if the heart's own impulses fail.

The capacity to recognize this problem and insert the necessary pacemaker is not found in all hospitals that otherwise take care of heart attack victims. Much depends on the ability of those diagnosing the initial situation to recognize the possible need of such pacing. Again, this represents a situation where the patient and/or his family —especially if coronary artery disease is known to be a problem—must assess the capacity of the hospital to which admission is anticipated. The easiest way to do this is to ask.

Third is *counterpulsation (mechanical assists).* The most dreaded complication of heart attacks is the development of mechanical failure—i.e., when the heart is damaged so badly that it cannot properly pump blood. Until recently the mortality for such situations has been almost 100 percent. One of the newer developments to cut down fatalities is the use of so-called "counterpulsation" devices to reduce the work load of a severely damaged heart. The technical details are beyond the scope of this discussion. Suffice it to say that this procedure requires highly trained personnel and sophisticated equipment; at present it is done only in major medical centers. It must also be said that such procedures are still experimental and far from being generally successful; they must still be described as "buying time" until bypass surgical procedures can be considered. But I mention them as a new approach to the desperate situation of the "pump failure" secondary to a heart attack—a situation which warrants desperate therapy.

Finally, a brief word about home care after a heart attack. I say brief because the only thing that can be said with certainty is that every heart attack victim must be treated individually—both medically and psychologically —following a heart attack. There are usually many questions to be answered concerning the activities of someone who has had a heart attack. This is one of those medical situations where a patient physician who will spend time with the victim and his family is invaluable. I wish I could say all physicians were adequate to this important task; some are not. A patient and/or family should never be embarrassed to ask even seemingly trivial questions; allaying anxiety is a very important part of the therapy of heart attack victims. So ask; with luck you will receive.

Risk Factors

Last, *but certainly not least,* I'd like to discuss the risk factors which have been pinpointed by prospective studies —most notably the famous Framingham, Massachusetts, studies. (Prospective studies are studies which are set up *before* the fact; they are constructed, with controls, to look at something as it develops rather than study old and possibly erroneous records.)

First, you should know that there is yet no hard statistical evidence to prove that elimination of risk factors will decrease the incidence of heart attacks and/or deaths from coronary artery disease. Studies are underway to establish proof, and a prudent attitude would be to avoid risk factors *without* such proof since waiting for proof may well be too late. You should also know that there is no proof that eliminating risk factors will halt or reverse coronary artery disease once it has begun. In other words, we do not know at what point in coronary artery disease the process of atherosclerosis becomes irreversible. Attention should really be devoted to our children from the moment of their birth—a "children's crusade," as the late heart specialist Dr. Paul Dudley White labeled such concern.

Having cast some doubt on the value of emphasizing risk factors, let me say that I fully expect this preventive approach to pay off—but I can't prove it. In the meantime, elimination of the risk factors is so sensible for other medical and social reasons that it is very much worth talking about.

Here is the list—and some comments.

1. *Heredity:* I'm talking now about heart attacks at an early age in close relatives—not about some distant appendages of the family tree who died at a ripe old age from some vague "heart failure." (After all, that's what does us all in ultimately.) But if there is a pattern of early heart attacks in parents or siblings or uncles and aunts—that is cause for concern. Two things should be done. First, since you can't do anything about your genes, even more attention must be paid to the risk factors you can do something about. And, second, you should be checked for evidence of some of

the more serious, genetically determined hyperlipidemias (increased blood fats) as described below.

2. *Hypertension:* Prevention of coronary artery disease and other heart disease is one of the many reasons for treating even mild elevations of blood pressure. Rather than repeat myself, I urge you to read the section on hypertension—and do it right now. (See page 309.)

3. *Smoking:* This is the one risk factor that is self-determined; we are not born with a cigarette in our mouth. Unfortunately, it is not as easy to stop as it is to start. People who smoke more than a pack a day have about a threefold increased risk of a heart attack. That should be motivation enough. If complete stopping is not possible, cutting down (under ten per day) is better than nothing. Next to heredity, smoking is probably the most important risk factor. (See page 353.)

4. *Diabetes:* Again, we face the fact that there is no evidence that control of diabetes will improve the outlook as far as heart disease is concerned. However, there are many other good reasons to control the disease (see page 272), and it certainly won't hurt the heart to do so.

5. *Increased blood fats:* The following is information about this complicated subject that everyone should have:

   • There are two major blood fats that we are concerned about in relation to heart disease, cholesterol and triglycerides. Depending on actual amounts of these two and other symptoms and signs, the diseases of blood fats—hyperlipidemias—are classified into five types, each with its own treatment. Therefore, *specific* diagnosis (requiring special blood tests taken after twelve to sixteen hours of fasting) and treatment is required—and this usually means the skills of an internist, cardiologist, or (for children) a competent pediatrician.

- Screening tests for cholesterol (which do not require fasting) are useful only as screening tests. Elevated cholesterol has a very strong predictive relationship to heart attacks. But, in order to determine the specific treatment of such elevation, more careful diagnosis with fasting blood tests must be done.
- Polyunsaturated fats tend to lower blood fats and should be used whenever possible. The use of animal foods rich in saturated fats (such as beef) should be minimized.
- If you are diagnosed as having elevated blood fats, your children should be checked to make sure they have not inherited the problem. The earlier the treatment, the better.

We now come to the more controversial risk factors—namely, obesity and exercise. Quite honestly, there is little hard evidence to implicate obesity *itself* (without associated hypertension, etc.) as a cause of heart disease. The same must be said of exercise—though there is some evidence to suggest that people who exercise regularly have a better chance of surviving a heart attack should they get one. On the other hand, there are plenty of other health and social reasons to exercise and to avoid obesity. Our instincts and observations tell us that people who exercise and maintain appropriate weight look better and feel better. One point should be made here: People who say they will not give up smoking because they will gain weight and that is bad for health are wrong. The tradeoff of excess weight for the stopping of smoking is a good one, medically. Ideally, one should accomplish both but, if a choice is necessary, stop the smoking and then attack any weight problem that develops.

A quick word about coffee—which was implicated as a risk factor by a recent Boston study. The results of that study have been criticized by others, and no other large study has supported those results. However, excess coffee drinking is ill advised in terms of general irritability.

In Summary

Coronary artery disease is this nation's No. 1 health problem; it kills more people in the prime of life than any other disease. We do not yet know the basic cause of coronary artery disease; support of basic research in this area is vital. In the meantime, we can all attempt to reduce the possibility of a heart attack in ourselves by paying attention to the risk factors I have described.

Rheumatic Heart Disease (*Rheumatic Fever*)

Because rheumatic heart disease is the most common cause of heart disease under age fifty, it merits a word of explanation. And the most important word in the context of this book is that the majority of rheumatic heart disease could be prevented with careful antibiotic eradication of strep infections—which is a backward way of saying that rheumatic heart disease is caused (the actual mechanism still not clear) by particular streptococcal bacteria usually one to four weeks after a strep infection of the upper respiratory tract (throat, ear).

When the strep bacteria affect the heart, they initiate the symptoms described as rheumatic fever. Actually, rheumatic fever must be described as a systemic (widespread) disease because it may affect organs other than the heart—particularly joints, skin, and lungs. But it is the effects on the heart that are the most worrisome. When acute rheumatic fever results in permanent damage to the heart, we speak of rheumatic heart disease to signify that the damage was caused initially by rheumatic fever.

The acute phase of rheumatic fever may be characterized by many symptoms including fever, joint pains (this combination of symptoms *always* merits investigation), skin changes and bumps, irregular body movements, etc. The actual diagnosis of rheumatic fever is based on a combination of documented findings from the history, physical exam, and laboratory tests. Once a diagnosis of rheumatic fever has been made, three periods of concern follow:

The acute phase (rheumatic fever) is the phase of the initial illness which is treated with antibiotics (penicillin is the drug of choice) and salicylates (of which aspirin is one form) and other measures as necessary. This initial phase may last months in children; it is usually shorter in adults. The death rate during this acute period is very low—one to two percent. The greater concern is whether permanent damage is done to the heart causing chronic rheumatic heart disease and this happens to some degree in a significant percent of rheumatic fever patients.

The chronic phase (rheumatic heart disease) may consist of anything from muscle damage resulting in heart failure to valvular disease of the heart resulting in their deformity and malfunction. Such disease may not become apparent until years after the acute rheumatic fever. When and if problems arise, a wide range of medical and surgical therapy may be appropriate under the direction of an internist–cardiologist. Most heart valve surgery is for damage from rheumatic heart disease.

The preventive phase is the third phase. The best prevention is the avoidance of strep infections when possible, though this is admittedly difficult. This is important for anyone who has ever had rheumatic fever since recurrent rheumatic fever increases the possibility of heart damage. Further aspects of prevention for the person who has had rheumatic fever or who has developed rheumatic heart disease include:

—Very prompt treatment with antibiotics for any possible strep throat infection.

—Continuous penicillin in low doses to prevent recurrences. The actual amounts and duration of such prophylaxis are determined on an individual basis.

—Special courses of antibiotics before any surgical procedure (including dental extractions) to minimize the possibility of developing other heart disease (endocarditis) on top of damaged heart valves from rheumatic heart disease.

All of this points up the careful counsel that must be given to victims of rheumatic fever and rheumatic heart disease. Anyone who has had these diseases must ask what can be done to minimize future problems.

In sum: rheumatic fever and rheumatic heart disease cut across many specialties—pediatricians (since rheumatic fever is most common in children between five and fifteen; internists–cardiologists (since heart disease is the most feared complication); heart surgeons (since many permanent valve deformities are subject to surgical correction). And the best treatment of this disease spectrum is the prompt treatment of strep infections. (See page 355.)

Heart Failure (*Congestive Heart Failure*)

I single this out as a separate heart disease because it is so common and so misunderstood. Actually, heart "failure" is not a separate disease in the sense of having a clearly defined single cause. It is, rather, the result of many possible underlying causes both within and without the heart. In fact, the three most common causes of heart failure are discussed in this book as separate diseases—hypertension, coronary artery disease, and rheumatic heart disease. Having made the point that heart failure is the result of other diseases, we are now prepared to define it as any situation in which the heart cannot keep up with the pumping demands upon it: It literally "fails" to do what is required.

Consider the three common causes listed above. In hypertension, the increased resistance against which the heart has to pump eventually causes the heart to enlarge (as the heart muscle tries to compensate) and wear out—resulting in failure as defined above. In coronary artery disease, resulting damage (including actual heart attacks) to the heart muscle because of poor blood supply again causes the weakened pump to fail to do its job. And, in rheumatic heart disease, valve damage causes improper and inefficient blood flow within the heart resulting in an eventually weakened heart that fails. There are many other possible causes of heart failure, but they all lead to the same situation.

That situation expresses itself in a common syndrome —a collection of symptoms and signs—that is called congestive heart failure. The word "congestive" is used because, when the pumping activity of the heart fails, the blood "backs up" in organs and vessels leading to the heart resulting in the "congestion" of those organs. In the lungs, this is expressed as difficulty breathing, waking up in the night short of breath, having to sleep with the head elevated on several pillows, etc. Other signs include elevated neck veins and an engorged, enlarged liver. In its severe, acute form, heart failure will cause the lungs to become filled with fluid—a condition described as "pulmonary edema"; this is a medical emergency and requires vigorous and prompt therapy.

It follows from what I have just said that treatment of heart failure must attempt to deal with the underlying cause (or causes) as well as the actual symptoms of failure. The basic therapy of failure itself involves many drugs and devices, depending on the severity of the failure. I would, however, like to mention two classes of drugs often used in the treatment of failure.

The first class is *digitalis*. Almost everyone has heard of this drug, since it is so commonly used in such a wide variety of heart problems. The name "digitalis" refers both to this class of drug and to one of the specific preparations; the most commonly used preparations are Digitoxin and Digoxin. Preparations differ in the amounts needed, times of onset, duration of action and rate of absorption. They all act to strengthen the contractions of the heart, and they all have important and potentially dangerous effects on the electrical conduction system of the heart. Indeed, the range between beneficial and dangerous (toxic) effects of digitalis is rather narrow, and careful attention by both patient and physician to warning signs of toxicity is necessary—slow rate, extra beats, nausea, headaches, fatigue, and, in more severe forms, diarrhea, confusion, blurring of vision. This is the main point I want to make: Digitalis, which is a great drug, can be dangerous if not taken carefully and exactly according to directions. One form cannot be substituted for another without careful direction by a knowledgeable physician. Never take someone else's "digitalis"; it may be an entirely different preparation. And contact your doctor at the *first* sign of trouble.

The second class is *diuretics*. These so-called "water-pills" are also widely used and misunderstood. There are many different preparations which have different mechanisms, all of which result in increased water loss through the urinary system. They too must be taken only under the careful direction of a physician. One special word of warning: These drugs generally promote potassium excretion in the urine, which may lead to decreased potassium levels in the blood—which in turn may lead to difficulty with heart action. Anyone taking diuretics for long periods of time should have his or her blood potassium levels checked periodically.

Heart failure, then, is caused by many diseases. Its treatment is directed both at the problems of the failure itself and, when possible, at the underlying cause. The drugs used in the treatment of congestive heart failure are potent and therefore potentially dangerous; they should never be taken without a physician's direction.

Palpitations

This term is used loosely by both doctors and lay persons to describe any unusual sensation of heart activity—rapid, forceful, or irregular beating. It is the most common patient complaint regarding the heart—and it is generally more frightening than dangerous.

The most common causes of the feelings described as palpitations are as follows:

1. *Sinus tachycardia:* This phrase means a rapid heartbeat (greater than 100 per minute) which is otherwise "normal" in terms of the conduction pattern on the electrocardiogram. I put "normal" in quotes because there may be an abnormal condition in the heart or elsewhere causing the rapid rate—for instance, anemia

secondary to gastrointestinal bleeding or an overactive thyroid gland. Actually, the vast majority of rapid heart rates are due to emotion—excitement, fear, nervousness. Careful examination and consequent reassurance are therefore usually the best medicine.

2. *Extra or early beats:* There are many technical phrases (e.g., premature ventricular systoles) to describe heartbeats which come early or are actually extra. The effect of such beats is often a sensation of the heart "skipping a beat," followed by an unusually strong "thumping" or "turning over" of the heart. The actual irregularity can usually be determined by careful bedside examination plus an electrocardiogram. The cause of such irregularity may or may not be related to real heart disease. Often it is not significant, particularly in the young.

3. *Paroxysmal atrial tachycardia:* This phenomenon is described as a rapid but regular "fluttering" which begins suddenly "out of the blue," lasts for minutes or hours and ends as suddenly as it began. It differs from sinus tachycardia in that the normal electrical conduction of the heart is temporarily abnormal. In an otherwise healthy person usually no other symptoms will be experienced—except fright. In older people or someone with underlying heart disease, fainting, chest pain, or difficulty breathing may be experienced. The most common causes of this phenomenon in someone without heart disease are emotional upsets, smoking, and excess coffee. Paroxysmal atrial tachycardia may signify heart disease, but this can usually be determined only with careful study.

To sum up, then, palpitations may or may not signify actual heart disease. When persistent or recurring, palpitations merit thorough investigation to rule out underlying and often correctable causes; such investigations are the province of a cardiologist. The majority of palpitations are not serious and require only understanding and reassurance. Often emotions are found to be the underlying culprit, and therapy will then lie in the direction of understanding, mild tranquilizers, and rearrangement of life-style when possible. Palpitations represent an instance where our bodies express our emotions in startling but usually not serious language.

From the above it is obvious that palpitations usually do not constitute a life-threatening emergency, even though the accompanying fright and ill-feeling warrants a visit to the emergency room. (Certainly if the palpitations are accompanied by other symptoms, such as chest pain, lightheadedness, or difficulty in breathing, they should be investigated immediately.) Usually the best source of therapy is a competent cardiologist who will make a thorough investigation to rule out serious causes and then take the time to explain carefully what is going on. This is one of those instances where patience is best for the patients.

Heart Murmurs

I have included this short section for one purpose: to point out that most heart murmurs, especially in childhood, are not serious. One of the tragedies of life is that person who has been labeled in childhood as "having a murmur" and has gone throughout life with unnecessary anxiety and limitation of activity.

Murmurs, which are sounds related to heart activity as heard through the stethoscope, can be divided into two categories. Most are "innocent" or "functional"—i.e., they do not signify disease. Some, of course, are signals of underlying disease—usually caused by abnormalities of valvular function or, in children, abnormalities of structure. In most cases, it is possible to say with certainty which category is applicable. Sometimes very sophisticated testing by a cardiologist in the hospital is necessary before a judgment can be made.

But, again, the purpose of this little squib is to warn against putting too much stock in the warning of a murmur made years ago to a person who since has felt and acted fine. In fact, many pediatricians are reluctant today to mention that they hear a murmur because they know it will cause unwarranted concern. Such silence is understandable, but it would probably be better to be complete in reporting findings but take the time to explain what is meant—or not meant. The fact of the matter is that most childhood murmurs disappear with time.

3

Lung Disease

A "good set of lungs" consists of three functional components. First are the *air passageways* leading from the back of the throat to a branching system to all parts of the lungs. The single trachea (windpipe) leads from the throat to a point in the middle of the chest, where it branches into two main tubes (the bronchi) which go to the lungs on each side of the chest. These two main tubes in turn branch into many smaller ones, which ultimately supply every small air sac in the lungs with air. These air passageways are often the site of infection (tracheitis, bronchitis, etc.), and the smaller ones may close down under several types of abnormal circumstances—asthma, for example.

The second component is *lung tissue,* which consists of 300 million microscopic air sacs (alveoli). Each one of these tiny sacs is surrounded by a small blood vessel, and it is at this microscopic level that the critical exchange of nutrient gas (oxygen) and waste gas (carbon dioxide) between the air we breathe and the bloodstream occurs. Anything that interferes with air getting into these sacs—

such as fluid in the lungs from pneumonia or heart failure —or with blood circulating through the lungs—such as a blood clot blocking lung circulation—threatens this exchange and therefore may threaten life.

Third are the *linings* surrounding the lungs on both sides of the chest. These linings (called "pleura") are very thin and double-layered; between the layers is a very thin film of fluid. Secondary to many conditions (infection, tumor, etc.), these linings become inflamed and produce excess fluid. Sometimes this condition—pleurisy—is very painful, especially with breathing movements, and sometimes the fluid accumulation is so extensive that it interferes with breathing and some of the fluid must be removed.

A technical distinction is sometimes made between *breathing* and *respiration*. The former refers to the mechanical act of air movement in and out of the lungs; the latter refers to the exchange of gases in the lungs and at the cellular level. In our discussions we will use the terms interchangeably in referring to the process by which we take oxygen and get rid of carbon dioxide.

Symptoms that we commonly think of in relation to lung disease—coughing, wheezing, etc.—may indeed be due to lung disease but may also be due to other problems (heart failure, anemia, aspiration of a foreign body, etc.). Persistent symptoms of this nature should not be passed off as "a little infection in my lungs" but should be investigated by a good primary care physician. Coughing up blood (hemoptysis) or any blood noticed in sputum always merits immediate investigation; usually such blood signifies nothing serious, but it may signify serious lung disease.

Finally a pitch against smoking: There is no single greater cause of ill health in general and lung disease in particular. We are exposed to enough air pollution without adding this intensive form of self-pollution. The section on Smoking in Part II discusses this point in greater detail (page 353).

Chronic Lung Disease (*Bronchitis and Emphysema*)

The terminology of this condition is confusing. The usual designation is COPE (chronic obstructive pulmonary emphysema) or COLD (chronic obstructive lung disease); I will use the term COPE. Whatever the terminology, the entity consists of (usually) slowly developing but irreversible damage to lung tissue resulting in poor gas exchange and the typical symptoms—constant shortness of breath made much worse by even minimal exertion and a chronic, often "productive" (containing pus) cough. The poor gas exchange results in hypoxemia (abnormally low blood oxygen levels), hypercapnia (abnormally high carbon dioxide levels), and acidosis; these abnormalities contribute to the weakness, lethargy, weight loss, etc., characteristic of more advanced forms of this condition. In final stages, this condition is marked by headache, impaired thought and confusion, asterixis (a jerking tremor of the hands), and an increasingly deep coma leading to death.

COPE has several possible causes, including the following:

1. *Long-term conditions affecting the air passages leading to the lungs:* That is why bronchitis (infection of the bronchi, the major tubes leading to each lung) is often included with emphysema (destruction of lung tissue itself) in a discussion of COPE. This precursor is not to be confused with isolated acute infections of

the air passages (referred to as "acute bronchitis"), which are self-limiting and/or successfully treated with appropriate medications. Recent evidence suggests that one of the effects of smoking is to cause partial constriction (closing) of some of the very small air passages (bronchioles), thereby leading to COPE. Other causes (such as occupational exposures—e.g., coal mining) of chronic bronchitis exist, but smoking is certainly the most serious and common cause.

2. Within the past ten years, association between emphysema and a deficiency of a certain protein (alpha-1-antitrypsin) has been well documented. This deficiency has been shown to be an inherited trait. The significance of this discovery lies in several possible areas, including *screening* programs that might allow couples to consider adoption instead of natural children (who would run a high risk of such disease if both parents were carriers of the gene for this deficiency) and *early identification* of persons with this deficiency to encourage avoidance of additional risk factors, such as smoking and urban pollution.

3. Many other disease entities can cause secondary chronic lung disease. Included in this list are silicosis, bronchiectasis (abcesses in the lung), etc.

This is one of those diseases where clearly the best treatment is prevention. Treatment of COPE is difficult and never fully successful. The disease is largely irreversible and usually continues to progress until the person afflicted dies in so-called "respiratory failure"—a euphemistic way of describing someone who dies gasping for air; this is a horrible, slow death. That's why I say that best treatment is prevention.

Prevention consists of avoiding irritants, and the most common irritant is inhaled cigarette smoke. One simple diagnostic test that can also be used by anyone now reading this page is as follows: Take a lighted wooden match and hold it six to twelve inches from your mouth. If you cannot blow this match out *with your mouth wide open* (without pursing your lips) you may be well on the way to the kind of lung disease described in this section. Throwing away your cigarettes and checking with a good primary care physician could be the two best moves you make in your lifetime. There are other factors to consider —urban air pollution, occupational exposures, and so on. But smoking is without question the most important cause and (except for lack of will power) the easiest to remove from the environment.

For someone suspected of developing COPE, there are many more sophisticated tests—pulmonary function tests —to pinpoint the exact stage or nature of disease. The point should be made that a normal chest X ray is no assurance that such disease is not developing; abnormal X rays mean extensive disease already exists.

Once actual disease exists, treatment becomes highly complex and must be tailored to the needs of the individual. More important than my outlining treatment possibilities is my pointing out that a good primary care physician with special training in pulmonary disease is the cornerstone of treatment; such treatment requires patient attention to details of the medical *and* psychological status of each person. And it is never too late to stop smoking as part of treatment. In early stages, much abnormal function is reversible; people are often amazed at how quickly they feel and function better if they stop smoking. And, even in advanced stages, stopping smoking will at least prevent further compromise of an already marginal breathing situation. Another important aspect of treatment is the prevention of infections in the bronchi and lungs. Often, persons with COPE are instructed in the use of antibiotics to be taken at the first sign of infection—fever, increasing cough, change in the look of the sputum, etc.

In summary, this disease, which is the most common, serious *chronic* disease in America, could be almost completely eliminated if we would retain our oral status as of birth—without cigarettes.

Pneumonia

Pneumonia means infection in the lungs. Such infection can be caused by many organisms—bacteria (pneumococcus is the most common), viruses, and organisms in between bacteria and viruses.

The earlier treatment is instituted, the better; this calls for early diagnosis. On the other hand, most "colds" do not lead to pneumonia and will get better without any treatment other than rest, fluids, and aspirin. This poses a dilemma for the person with a cold: When is the time to get it checked out? There are no firm rules, but the presence of any of the following suggests more strongly the possibility of pneumonia:

1. Fever greater than 102° orally

2. Pain in the chest, either constant or associated with breathing

3. Coughing of sputum which is thick, greenish, yellow, or blood-tinged (so-called "productive" sputum).

4. So-called "shaking chills" associated with high fever and sweats

A quick word about "atypical" pneumonias. This term is applied to pneumonias caused by viruses or other organisms than bacteria. (This kind of pneumonia has other names—Eaton's agent pneumonia, mycoplasmal pneumonia, primary atypical pneumonia.) The point to be made is that, while this kind of pneumonia is usually associated with less fever and fewer symptoms, it can often lay the victim low for a prolonged period of time; death, however, is rare. X-ray abnormalities often persist for months, even though the patient feels better in weeks. Broad spectrum antibiotics (tetracycline, erythromycin, and so on) are often used to treat this kind of pneumonia.

Penicillin is still the most common and effective drug for treatment of bacterial pneumonia, since more than eighty percent of pneumonias are caused by the pneumococcal bacterium, which is very sensitive to penicillin. In young, otherwise healthy persons with mild pneumonias, home treatment with oral antibiotics is usually possible. Conversely, in older people or persons with other disease, hospitalization for treatment with intravenous antibiotics is often needed.

Finally, reading of the section on Infectious Disease would be useful (see page 187).

Lung Cancer

Only five percent (five!) of patients with lung cancer are alive five years after the disease was first diagnosed. That is the story of lung cancer in a nutshell.

If ever prevention was the cure, it is true of this terrible disease. And prevention means just what the signs say: NO SMOKING. It is true that there may be other contributing causes. It is true that we don't know the final causative link between smoking and lung cancer. But it is also true that heavy cigarette smokers have a *twenty-three times greater* chance of getting lung cancer than the nonsmoker. And it is also true that nonsmokers rarely get lung cancer.

Early diagnosis offers the only hope of cure; surgical removal of the small tumors before they spread is the only successful, curative treatment. The problem is that we have no reliable method of early detection for lung cancer. The yearly chest X ray, while recommended as better than nothing for the heavy smoker over forty, is really that—better than nothing, but not much better. There are other techniques of diagnosis: sputum cytology, bronchoscopy, node biopsy, needle aspiration, mediastinoscopy, etc. When these fancy techniques are used, however, it usually means that if something is found it is too late.

Tuberculosis

The most important point to be made about this disease is that *it is still around*. Too many people assume that TB is a disease of the past. While it is true that TB can now be successfully treated in the vast majority of cases and is therefore no longer the great scourge of the past, the actual incidence of TB is still significant and represents a major public health problem.

In the context of this book, the following summary points concerning TB should suffice:

1. The initial symptoms of TB are so many and frequently so subtle that early diagnosis is often difficult. While the yearly chest X ray is no longer recommended routinely for everyone, it is useful in certain high-risk persons—including those with a history of

TB or close contacts with persons with TB, those with a positive skin test in the past, those working in a high-risk environment (hospital workers, etc.), and those with certain other high-risk conditions such as silicosis, diabetes, and alcoholism.

2. The "skin test" remains the best screening test available. There are several different kinds of skin tests, but the most accurate is the intradermal (a needle stuck in the superficial layer of the skin) test performed with Tween-80 stabilized PPD (I list that technical information in case you have reason to be concerned about the accuracy of your skin test). Once a skin test is positive it remains positive for life and follow-up screening should consist of at least yearly chest X rays; skin tests should not be done on persons with known active disease or past positive tests.

3. In the situation where a skin test changes from known past negative tests to a positive test, two considerations become important. First, a thorough search must be made to rule out active disease. (A positive skin test does not mean contagious tuberculosis; it implies exposure to the disease sometime in the past. A change from negative to positive implies exposure during the time since the last negative test). If active disease is found, it must be treated (for one to three years) with the excellent drugs now available. If no active disease is found, the question of prophylactic drug therapy must be faced. Most authorities still recommend that "converters" (persons whose skin tests have recently changed from known negative to positive) who are under age thirty-five or anyone with certain other diseases (such as diabetes) be treated with a one-year course of INH. However, some authorities are concerned about

the possible toxic effects of this drug and prefer to follow the patient closely instead and await signs of active disease before treatment. The good advice of a competent physician is the only "rule" I can offer on this one.

4. The person who does have active TB is "safe" as long as he or she is under good medical care and taking antituberculous drugs as prescribed. I mention this because too many TB patients have become outcasts in the eyes of family and friends and this is totally unwarranted *if* the person is being cared for adequately. Certainly a new case of TB must be isolated until it is under adequate treatment (several days to weeks), and all the close contacts of such a person must be carefully examined for evidence of TB. But once under treatment strong family support is helpful and medically safe.

Finally, I plug for skin-testing (and chest X rays in those with positive skin tests). A TB skin test should be part of any physical exam—unless there is definite knowledge of a previously positive skin test, in which case a chest X ray is in order. Skin tests should be done by the pediatrician periodically and continue throughout life.

4

Cancer

This section represents a general introduction to the subject of cancer; specific cancers are discussed in appropriate sections throughout the book.

Few words have the emotional impact of the word "cancer." Our society is not the first to attach ugly and frightening images to the word. The ancient Greeks thought that spreading, cancerous growths resembled the claws of a crab; they called it "the crablike disease," *karkinos,* the Latin translation of which is *cancer.* Most of us regard the diagnosis of cancer as an automatic death sentence. The facts of the matter, however, are these:

- *Of the more than half-million persons with newly diagnosed cancer each year, one-third will be permanently cured; many others will lead a normal life for many fruitful years.*

- *Of those who die each year from cancer, it is estimated that over 100,000 of them will have died needlessly because of late diagnosis and inadequate treatment.*

- *While it is true that certain cancers—such as stomach and lung cancers—are very difficult to diagnose early and treat effectively, other very common cancers can be detected early and often treated successfully. Included in this group are cancers of the bowel, cancer of the cervix and uterus, and breast cancer. Also included in this group of curable cancers are mouth cancers, skin cancers (the most common cancer of all), cancers of the kidney and of the urinary system, cancers of the prostate, and many other types.*

It is absolutely essential to understand that cancer is not one but many diseases which can differ markedly in causes, methods of diagnosis, and treatments. However, all cancers *do* share one common feature: They all represent abnormal cells growing out of control. The cells of a cancerous growth are irregular in size and shape. They do not form useful tissues or organs and they do not stop multiplying. Masses of these abnormal cells sooner or later result in a lump or swelling called a tumor. A mass of cells that shows little deviation from normal and only limited penetration into the surrounding area with no spread to other areas is called a benign tumor. A growth of cells which is markedly abnormal in structure and which penetrates and spreads is a malignant tumor, or what we commonly describe as cancer.

Now we're ready to ask the $64 billion question. Why does normal cell growth go berserk? Some answers may come from the science of immunology, which deals with the way the body manages to fight everything that is not a normal part of us. For example, our bodies protect themselves against foreign invaders like bacteria and viruses by producing antibodies which destroy such foreign tissue. So the immunologists are asking this intriguing question: Could it be that this same immune system fights abnormal cells and that cancer is the result of a breakdown in our immunological defenses? In other words, rather than concentrating on why so many people get cancer, maybe we should be asking why *most* people *don't* get cancer. (One example of this kind of thinking is the use of a tuberculosis vaccine, BGG, to "turn on" the immunology system of a cancer patient; though this kind of treatment is still experimental there is evidence that it may be effective in some cancers.)

Until answers to these basic questions are found, the name of the game is still early detection. Specific information on early detection will be found in appropriate sections throughout the book. The American Cancer Society's seven warning signs are precisely that—warnings of possible danger which, if taken as early signals, may lead to early detection and cure. These warning signs may be summarized by saying that any persistent (more than a few days) change in body *appearance* (sores, warts, lumps, thickenings) or *function* (unusual bleeding or discharge, change in bowel or bladder habits, indigestion or difficulty in swallowing, nagging cough or hoarseness) *must* be investigated under the direction of a physician.

I've commented on several areas of cancer but as yet have said nothing about causes. Partly that's because "cancer" is, as I've said, many diseases with many possible causes; it seems unlikely that there is a single cause or will be a single cure. But there are some things we do know, that you should know.

For example, we know that familial tendencies do occur in certain cancers. If there is a family history of cancer, you should consult with your doctor as to whether any particular checks are in order for you. For example, any woman with a mother or sister who has had breast cancer should pay particular attention to careful monthly examinations and yearly checkups, including mammograms, which are special X-ray screening studies now proving to be very useful in early detection.

A word about viruses is in order. You should understand that the viruses which are being studied in relationship to cancer are not the same viruses we associate with infection. In other words, they are not contagious, as are the viruses of the common cold, for example. As yet, there is no definite proof that viruses cause human cancer, but there is great interest in this line of research.

There are, however, some factors which are so frequently associated with a given cancer that we must speak of them as causes, even though we may not know the exact way in which they cause the cancer. Certain chemicals (vinyl chloride, for example) are known to be carcinogenic, that is, cancer causing. We are very much dependent on government and private surveillance to detect such harmful substances. In the meantime, each of us should question the appropriate authorities concerning substances to which we might be constantly exposed in our work or activity.

Chronic irritation is another cause of cancer. Any kind of constant irritation to tissues is a possible cause of cancer, but the classic example is chronic overexposure to sunlight leading to skin cancer. Skin cancer is high on the list of curable cancers—but 5000 people a year do die from it.

Finally, and most significantly, smoking causes lung cancer. If you are over forty and have smoked two packs a day for ten years or more, your chances are twenty-three times greater of getting lung cancer than the nonsmoker. Lung cancer will strike almost 100,000 men and women this year and kill more than ninety percent of these people. Lung cancer is very difficult to diagnose early; it is already hopeless in almost ninety-five percent of its victims at the time of first diagnosis. Yearly chest X rays offer little protection. Smoking may not be the only cause of lung cancer, but it is so clearly the major cause that others are not worth talking about—period.

Finally, a quick word about treatment. Basically, all cancer treatment involves one of three kinds of therapy.

1. *Surgery* is the most dramatic and generally offers the best chance of cure if detection is early. Great progress has been made in the care of the surgical patient and many operations which were daring ten years ago are routine today.

2. *Radiation therapy* is based on the fact that cancerous cells are often more susceptible to destruction by high voltage radiation than normal cells. Some cancers—certain tumors of the testicles, for example—are very responsive to radiotherapy and may be treated solely with radiation.

3. *Chemotherapy,* a fancy word for treatment with cancer drugs, is an area of intensive investigation and rapidly changing knowledge. Drug therapy offers some real success stories; some forms of leukemia, for example, can now be "cured" with drug therapy. Such drug therapy often involves careful orchestration of multiple drugs, with attention to difficult side effects.

Indeed, treatment for cancer may involve any or all of these methods in a combination of approaches requiring scientific knowledge and clinical experience of the highest order. Which leads me to say this: The most important point I can make about the diagnosis and treatment of

cancer in this book concerns the source of treatment—
whom to see and *where* to go.

Cancer treatment today has become so complex that it
requires the combined skills of many specialists working
together in a hospital with modern diagnostic and treatment equipment. The obvious problem is to know how
to find such an environment. Notice the emphasis on
knowing and *finding*. Hard thinking and work are required;
this is no time for blind loyalty to the doctor who has
seen your family through countless bouts of the flu. This
is not to say that your doctors and your hospital are inadequate. But you and your family, when and if afflicted
with cancer, must not assume adequacy; you must ask
and question. Here is a good checklist:

- *Does your doctor have special training in the area
  of treatment being proposed? In other words (and
  you can use these words), is he a "cancer specialist?"
  Aside from the oncologist—the cancer specialist of
  internal medicine—there are no formal designations for cancer specialists. But surgeons, gynecologists, pediatricians, radiologists—all have special
  opportunities for training in cancer treatment, and
  you should ask about them.*

- *How much experience has your doctor had in the
  kind of cancer you are concerned about? There are
  no easy guidelines, but one or two cases of a given
  kind a year hardly qualifies as extensive experience.
  You should ask about experience.*

- *What kind of expertise does your hospital have in
  dealing with cancer? Does it have a tumor committee composed of specialists in all areas of cancer
  treatment who together review cancer cases? Does*

*it have a tumor registry or some comparable method
of keeping track of treatment statistics? Does it have
available as consultants outstanding specialists in
the cases that require very special and up-to-date
knowledge?*

All of this is not to frighten you but to lay it on the line:
It is your body and your life. You have every right to ask
and to know.

One final source of information is worth mentioning—
the National Cancer Institute, commonly called the NCI,
a part of the National Institutes of Health in Bethesda,
Maryland. The NCI offers free mail advice as to sources
of treatment expertise. When in doubt, a letter to the
following address might be helpful: Office of Cancer Com-
munications, Building 31, Room 10-A-23, National Cancer
Institute, Bethesda, Md. 20014. Individualized replies are
sent within two weeks.

5

Gastrointestinal (GI) Disease

No part of us is more responsive to our emotions than our digestive organs. When we talk about "feeling it in my guts" we are not just being figurative. Rare is the individual who has not experienced sudden defecation or regurgitation (otherwise known as diarrhea or vomiting) in response to emotional stimuli. Often, less pronounced changes exist for longer periods without explanation. The big problem, however, is that any one of these common complaints *may* also be a sign of serious disease. To sort out the "real" from the "functional" is a challenge to both patient and physician.

The gastrointestinal (hereafter referred to as GI) system includes all structures in the "tube" leading from mouth to anus plus several important organs that attach to the GI tract—including the liver, gall bladder, and pancreas. The medical specialist in GI diseases is called a gastroenterologist—or more commonly a GI specialist; such a doctor has had basic training in general internal medicine plus extra training in GI diseases. Most well-trained primary care physicians are also competent to handle GI problems. You should go to these *nonsurgical* doctors first with any GI complaint short of an obvious emergency such as severe pain or massive loss of blood from either end of the GI tract. I say this simply because the nonsurgeon is more likely to try to avoid surgery. This is not just a matter of "unnecessary surgery" but an understandable orientation of training and medical bias. A surgeon, however, becomes absolutely essential whenever an "acute abdomen" (which I will define shortly) is part of the picture; in such cases, no delay should occur in seeking the advice of a surgeon.

Since the phrase "acute abdomen" is often used by medical persons, it merits explanation in this discussion. The phrase refers to signs from the physical examination (extreme tenderness, rigid muscles, marked changes in bowel sounds as heard through the stethoscope, etc.) which add up to a picture of something potentially catastrophic going on inside the abdomen. Such a situation means surgery is likely to be required and that a surgeon should be consulted promptly. When the examination does not add up to such a picture, however, there is more time for studies and the adoption of a "wait and see" attitude. I take time to outline this basic distinction because many people with severe pain feel that surgery is the answer and cannot understand why a doctor sometimes seems willing to proceed more cautiously. Another point of misunderstanding by patients is the withholding of pain medication in certain cases of abdominal pain. When a physician does this he is appropriately using pain as one of the best indicators of what is going on inside the abdomen; strong pain medication would wipe out this indicator, and (for example) a sudden rupture inside the abdomen might occur without being heralded by a sudden increase in pain.

X-ray studies are still the mainstay of GI diagnosis. However, many new techniques of diagnosis are available to the trained specialist. The most important of these is probably *endoscopy*—the insertion of a tube into the appropriate opening (mouth or anus) for a direct look at the possible problem—bleeding site, ulcer, cancer, inflammation, etc. There are several different types of endoscopes, the newest being flexible fiberoptic "scopes" allowing more extensive examination. The obvious point of such examination is better diagnosis than can be provided by barium X ray without resorting to surgical exploration. Such examinations are done by both gastroenterologists and surgeons.

A special word about the sigmoidoscope is in order since it is still the most commonly used endoscope. The sigmoidoscope is a rigid, hollow instrument (referred to by medical people somewhat sadistically as "the silver bullet") which can be inserted through the anus to a distance of about ten inches into the end part of the large intestine called the sigmoid—hence the name. The significance of the procedure of sigmoidoscopy lies in the following:

1. It is a simple procedure which involves some discomfort for the patient but which can be done in minutes in an office setting. In other words, its widespread use is feasible. Both primary care and specialist physicians are trained to use it.

2. Many cancers of the colon are within the range of the sigmoidoscope, making it very useful in the investigation of any suspicious symptoms of colon cancer.

3. Many other abnormalities of the colon (such as polyps and colitis) can be seen via the sigmoidoscope. Also, tissue specimens can sometimes be "biopsied" through this instrument, thus avoiding surgery.

Next a comment about the most common of GI complaints—nausea, vomiting, and diarrhea, the "GI blahs." What was said about GI symptoms in the first paragraph is eminently true of this infamous triad; they may signify serious disease but most often they reflect less serious and temporary upsets, usually a GI viral infection referred to as "viral gastroenteritis." The actual diagnosis of viral gastroenteritis is usually one of exclusion. In other words, if, after careful examination, there is no strong evidence to suggest more localized disease (such as appendicitis or an ulcer), the conclusion is that it is a general GI upset most likely caused by a virus. Such a condition, though causing the individual afflicted to feel absolutely miserable, usually clears in twenty-four to seventy-two hours without treatment other than restricted diet and medications for severe vomiting and/or diarrhea.

Finally, a word about cancers of the GI tract. Unfortunately, some cancers of the GI tract are difficult to diagnose early enough for surgical cure; this includes most cancers of the esophagus, stomach, *small* intestine (rare), pancreas, and gall bladder. However, cancers of the large intestine (colon and rectum) are much more amenable to diagnosis and cure, so I am devoting a separate section to them. Certainly any persistent change in bowel habits, *any* evidence of bleeding from the GI tract, or any other persistent symptoms should be investigated to make sure that a curable GI cancer is not the cause. And, as will be stressed in the section on colon and rectal cancer, a rectal exam (including a test for hidden blood) should be a part of any physical exam done past age forty.

Now, on to some specific GI problems.

Appendicitis

This common disease warrants discussion for two reasons: (1). Some persons still wait too long in seeking attention for appendicitis, thereby increasing the chances of rupture. (2). The "wait and see" attitude of physicians is often misunderstood by understandably concerned parents.

Though the development of appendicitis is usually described as a "classical" progression from generalized upper abdominal pain accompanied by nausea to localized right lower abdominal pain within two to twelve hours, the fact is that almost anything can happen in appendicitis, and it can be particularly confusing in the very young and elderly. Thus, any new and persistent (lasting more than a few hours) abdominal distress must be checked out.

Having aroused such concern, I will now proceed to state that often appendicitis cannot be diagnosed in the early stages and therefore the physician will advise "careful watching" for twelve to twenty-four hours. So why go early? Two reasons: (1). Certain baseline physical and laboratory values can be established for comparison should trouble persist or increase. (2). The more rapidly developing case (which would lead more rapidly to perforation) will not be missed.

A thorough examination for appendicitis involves careful examination of the abdomen, the checking of blood and urine samples, *and* a rectal (plus a possible pelvic in the female) examination. The tender and inflamed appendix is near the rectum, so a rectal exam is therefore often useful in establishing the diagnosis.

In many cases, a diagnosis of appendicitis can be established at the first examination and surgery can be definitely recommended. (If sufficient symptoms exist, this is one of those instances where it pays to err on the side of "unnecessary" surgery since the risk of surgery is so small and the dangers of a ruptured appendix are comparatively much greater.) But quite often the advice of the examining physician will be to "watch for the next twenty-four hours," either at home or in the hospital. Such advice is not unreasonable, because, if it is appendicitis, the trouble will not go away and will indeed get worse; on the other hand, transient "gastroenteritis" will improve during this time and surgery can be avoided.

Cancer of the Colon and Rectum

Cancer of the large intestine (the colon and the rectum, which is the end part of the large intestine) kills more people than any other cancer except lung cancer. It's worth knowing about—particularly because this is a cancer that offers a good chance of cure if certain warning signs are heeded and if routine rectal exams are done past age forty.

You should know the following about this cancer:

1. Many cancers of the rectum are within reach of a rectal finger exam. Therefore—and I can't say it too often—this simple procedure (including a test for hidden blood) should be done as part of any physical examination in both men and women. If there are *any* symptoms of possible cancer (see below), a sigmoidoscopic exam is also a must.

2. Any *persistent* change in bowel habit should be investigated. The obvious question is: What is persistent? Let's be arbitrary: Any change in customary bowel habit (whether the change be constipation or looseness) that lasts for more than one week merits investigation. Most such situations turn out *not* to be cancer, but the chance is not worth taking.

3. *Any* bleeding from the rectum should be investigated. Most such bleeding is *not* cancer, but is usually due to hemorrhoids. Again, however, the chance is not worth taking. The real problem comes for someone who knows he has hemorrhoids; such a person understandably attributes any bleeding to his known hemorrhoids. This is the only exception I dare make: If bleeding from hemorrhoids has been *recently* established, one might wait a few days if bleeding—and I'm obviously talking about bleeding in small amounts —occurs before rechecking.

Two questions are worth discussing. One is whether polyps (growths of the inner surface of the colon) are cancerous. This is an important question, because polyps are often found coincidentally in barium enema X rays done for other reasons and then the question of what to do arises. If the polyp is on a long stalk (pedunculated) and its diameter is less than 1.0 cm., its chances of being cancerous are small; periodic followup observation via yearly X rays is a reasonable approach. If, however, the polyp is flat (sessile) or large its chances of being cancerous are greater; these should be removed. If the surgeon involved can remove polyps through a scope inserted via the rectum, that is acceptable; in some cases, however, distribution and appearance of polyps make abdominal surgery more advisable. Polyps represent an area where judgment still must be exercised and a second opinion may well be in order.

Another question concerns the role of diet in the cause of colonic cancer (and other GI problems). Dr. Burkitt (who has done extensive study of diseases in Africa) has called attention to the possible correlation between decreased roughage in the diet and an increased incidence of colonic cancer. While this correlation is not firmly proven and while diet is certainly not the only "relationship" in cancer of the colon, it would seem a relatively simple matter to include more roughage (vegetables, unprocessed cereals, bran, etc.) in our diets until evidence becomes clearer.

Finally, a word about colostomies (a connection of the colon to the abdominal wall, with collection of feces in a bag), since this is often the result of surgery for cancer of the end part of the colon or rectum. This word usually strikes distaste if not fear in the hearer. That's an understandable reaction, but the care of colostomies today is much easier and better understood than twenty years ago, and the vast majority of people with them can lead a *completely* normal life in terms of activity—including swimming and sex and everything in between. There are special clinics which help people adjust to colostomies and teach them how to use the superb equipment that is now available.

Diverticulosis and Diverticulitis

A diverticulum is a "pouch or pocket leading from a main cavity or tube." Diverticula (plural) of the large intestine can occur at any age, but become increasingly common after age forty; by the time of age eighty, most of the population would demonstrate such outpouchings on barium enema X rays. When such outpouchings are seen on X ray (often coincidental to other more important findings), the condition is described as diverticulosis. Only when these outpouchings become inflamed is the situation described as Diverticulitis; this happens in only a small num-

ber of all persons with diverticula, but, since the outpouchings are so common, diverticulitis is a common
medical problem.

Diverticulitis is often described as "left-sided appendicitis," since the pain is often felt in the lower left part of
the abdomen. Like appendicitis, however, the manifestations of diverticulitis can be manifold and subtle. Very
occasionally, after careful study, exploratory surgery will
be necessary to decide the issue; this is particularly true
when X-ray appearance and even endoscopic exam (sticking a tube up via the rectum for a direct look) cannot
make the distinction between cancer of the colon and
diverticulitis. In such cases, exploratory ("looking for an
answer") surgery is quite justified.

In most cases, treatment of diverticulitis does not require surgery. There is some controversy as to the best diet
for people with diverticula, and recommendations seem
to change every few years; the current recommendation
is a high residue (bulky) diet without small hard things
such as nuts or seeds. Probably the most important part
of therapy—except for antibiotics in acute inflammation
—is to avoid constipation in the easiest and most certain
way; prunes are always a good place to start, but more
than that may be required.

Surgery does become legitimate in addition to the
diagnostic situation described above, for complications—
uncontrollable bleeding, abscess formations, rupture, etc.
Careful teamwork between the nonsurgical physician and
the surgeon is essential, especially since diverticulitis patients are often older and therefore greater surgical risks.

Finally, returning to the distinction described in the
first paragraph, don't worry about your "tics" (as doctors
often refer to them) unless they give you trouble. Too
many people have been informed about their X-ray find-

ings of diverticula only to worry unnecessarily; remember, the great majority of them never act up.

Gall Bladder Disease

Unlike the appendix, the gall bladder serves a function—namely, the storage of bile from the liver (to be released when appropriate to aid in digesting food). Like the appendix, however, the gall bladder is not essential to life. (Like the appendix, it *is* essential to the incomes of many surgeons.)

For those few of you who like tongue twisters, I'll list the following terms:

1. *Cholecystitis:* Inflammation of the gall bladder, usually, but not always, caused by . . .

2. *Cholelithiasis:* Stones in the gall bladder, which may also be found in the duct leading from the gall bladder to the small intestine, in which case it is called . . .

3. *Choledocholithiasis:* Stones in the duct system.

(If you can say each of those three times fast, you can move on!)

Thus, when we speak of "gall bladder disease" we are usually speaking of stones in the gall bladder or its ducts causing inflammation and resulting in right upper quadrant pain, nausea, and vomiting—usually following eating.

There are several important questions relating to gallstone disease. First, it must be stressed that not all "indigestion following foods" is due to gallstones. It is imperative that X-ray studies (involving the taking of oral tablets and/or the injection of intravenous dye) confirm gallstones and/or a nonfunctioning gall bladder as the cause of symptoms. Too many operations to remove a gall bladder (*cholecystectomy*—I didn't have the heart to add that to the list above) have been done without proving that the gall bladder was the culprit; the result of such ill-advised surgery is a patient with a scar, a bill, and persistent symptoms. If X-ray studies do demonstrate gall bladder disease consistent with stones, surgery is the answer, assuming the patient can tolerate major surgery. Generally, surgery is not advised during an acute attack unless perforation or gangrene are suspected. Rather, the patient is treated conservatively to get the attack under control and surgery is scheduled several weeks later. However, many surgeons are operating earlier in cases where the diagnosis is without question; results of such surgery in good-risk patients appear to be good.

One question often asked is this: What should be done about gallstones found accidentally during routine or other X-ray studies (so-called "silent" stones)? There is disagreement on this one, but most would say that surgery is not advisable until symptoms have occurred—except in diabetics, who are at higher risk of developing complications from gall bladder disease. (Autopsy studies indicate that, by age eighty, forty percent of people have developed gallstones; most of them did not need surgery and died of something other than gall bladder disease.) Once symptoms occur, removal of the gall bladder under elective (nonacute, nonemergency) conditions is clearly advisable versus waiting for continuing attacks during which surgery, if required, is more dangerous.

Another question concerns the treatment of gallstones with pills which "dissolve" gallstones. This is an issue under active investigation since first reported by the Mayo Clinic several years ago. The present status of such treatment is still considered experimental, since side-effects and long-range effects have not been fully evaluated; the pills are not available for general use. Though such treatment does not work for all kinds of gallstones, the continuing evidence is that such pills do indeed dissolve many stones over a period of months and years. Pills will not be the answer in every case, but the evidence to date makes continued study definitely worthwhile.

Finally, a reminder again that not all "indigestion" is due to gallstones. This becomes important to stress to the individual who has had stones demonstrated on X ray and then assumes all future digestive difficulties are due to "the stones." Any persistent digestive difficulty should be investigated. It may be the stones (in which case surgery should be considered), but it may not be.

Heartburn (*Reflux Esophagitis*) and Hiatus Hernia

These two topics tie together in most people's minds though there are many possible causes of "heartburn" besides Hiatus Hernia. Most serious of the other causes of heartburn is the pain or discomfort of true *heart pain*—pain due to ischemic heart disease (page 121). However, most heartburn is secondary to disturbances in the GI tract near enough to the heart to be felt in the general area of the lower chest. The most common GI cause of "heartburn" is reflux of acid from the stomach into the esophagus.

The food pipe (esophagus) from the throat to the stomach enters the abdominal cavity via an opening—or hiatus—in the diaphragm which separates the chest from the abdominal cavity. Since the term hernia means "the protrusion of an organ or tissue through an abnormal opening," you can see that "hiatus hernia" refers to conditions in which part of the stomach pushes up through the diaphragm into the lower part of the chest. (There are several different types of such hernia, but for our purposes the above description is sufficient.)

So far, so good. The problem is, however, that such an anatomical defect demonstrated on an X ray does not prove that it is the source of symptoms—and vice versa. It has been estimated that a hiatus hernia could be demonstrated by careful X-ray study in the majority of persons over sixty; most, fortunately, would have no symptoms and would not otherwise know they had such an anatomical problem. On the other hand, persons with classical symptoms of "heartburn" may not demonstrate the abnormal anatomy even with repeated careful X-ray exam— which involves swallowing barium with the patient in several positions, including the head and trunk tipped down.

All of which is to say that more than the deranged anatomy of hiatus hernia is required to cause the symptoms of heartburn. What is required is *reflux*—the "upstream" passage of stomach acid (and more rarely, bile) into the esophagus, which is not built to resist such juices. When these juices produce symptoms of "burning" (or "heartburn"), the condition is described as *reflux esophagitis*. There are several studies which attempt to relate symptoms of "heartburn" to reflux; probably the best of these is the measurement of increased acidity in the lower part of the esophagus after instilling some acid into the stomach. Such proof of reflux from the stomach into the esophagus demonstrates a functional breakdown of the normal pressure zone between the esophagus and stomach whether or not an actual anatomical defect such as a hiatus hernia exists.

The reason I have spent so much time making these points is to make the following point: Surgery to correct a hiatus hernia (as demonstrated on X ray) should never be performed *unless* symptoms have been clearly related to reflux which has not been responsive to medical therapy. More than ninety percent of patients with reflux esophagitis can be managed by nonsurgical treatment— reduction in weight, avoidance of body positions which encourage reflux (the reason for blocks to elevate the head of the bed at night), eating smaller amounts of food at any given time, antacids, etc. When such treatment fails or when complications of esophagitis arise, surgery may be necessary. The surgical procedures used involve correction of any hernia and a revision of the junction between the lower end of the esophagus and the stomach to decrease reflux.

Obviously a competent primary care physician (in this case, preferably a gastroenterologist) should be consulted before surgery "to correct a hiatus hernia" is done. One of his roles as a nonsurgeon is to make sure that symptoms are due to reflux esophagitis and that adequate medical treatment has been tried.

Inflammatory Bowel Disease (*Versus "Irritable Colon" and "Gastritis"*)

The terminology of conditions affecting the intestines is confusing and often used loosely by both physicians and lay people. Since true inflammatory disease of the intestines (disease marked by inflammatory changes in the lining of the intestines) may have serious implications, it is important to separate such disease from functional conditions (without demonstrable changes in anatomy) which are less serious. The two major inflammatory diseases you might hear about are these:

1. *Ulcerative colitis (chronic nonspecific ulcerative colitis):* This disease affects the *large* intestine (colon) producing bloody diarrhea, abdominal pain, fever, weight loss, and possible disease in other parts of the body—including arthritis, skin disorders, eye inflammation, etc.

2. *Regional enteritis:* This disease affects the *small* intestine, producing many types of GI distress (depending on the extent and location of the disease). Like ulcerative colitis, the disease can cause general debility and often produces symptoms elsewhere in the body. (Regional enteritis is sometimes referred to as "Crohn's disease," and a similar type of inflammation may affect the large intestine, in which case it is described as "Crohn's disease of the colon.")

I spend this time on terminology because, unfortunately, many people have the idea that they have "colitis" because somewhere along the line they have been told that their colon is "irritable" or that they have a "touch of colitis." Since true ulcerative colitis (as described above) is often a serious disease, such confusion may be worrisome. Many people who think they have "colitis" have what is more appropriately described as the "irritable colon syndrome." This syndrome has also been referred to as "spastic colitis," "mucous colitis," "unstable colon," and so on. All of these terms reflect some of the possible functional disturbances that can occur in people who are "uptight" about life in general and their bowel function in particular; the most typical combination of symptoms is that of abdominal cramps combined with the difficult passage of small-caliber stools. This condition should be thoroughly investigated to rule out other more serious diseases of the intestines. But when, in fact, no real pathology can be demonstrated, attention to the total personality of the person with these complaints is crucial.

Like "colitis," the term "gastritis" is often used for GI symptoms for which no other diagnosis can be made. The specific diagnosis of gastritis (inflammation of the lining of the stomach) can only be made from a tissue specimen (obtained via surgery or endoscopy) and examined under the microscope. This is done only for a patient with persistently troublesome symptoms. The more common situation is for an acute attack of nausea and vomiting to be caused by something—irritants such as alcohol, viruses, or bacteria—that will clear with time and conservative treatment. Such a diagnosis and course of treatment, however, can only be entertained after careful examination to rule out more specifically treatable conditions—ulcer, appendicitis, etc. Therefore I feel strongly that everyone with new and more than mild symptoms must be seen in person—not just diagnosed over a telephone—by a physician at least once. I know some will argue with me—especially busy pediatricians in the midst of a viral gastroenteritis epidemic—but I must state my opinion as I believe it.

The inflammatory bowel diseases (ulcerative colitis and regional enteritis) require very intensive treatment; usually the special skills of a gastroenterologist are required. An especially important consideration in both diseases is the role of surgery; great judgment is required as to the timing and extent of surgery. Also, these diseases usually are accompanied by significant psychological upset requiring a sympathetic physician–patient relationship.

Liver Disease (*Hepatitis, Cirrhosis, and Alcoholic Liver Disease*)

Our livers are among those things in life that we take for granted until they cause trouble. Most people have little appreciation for the complexity of the function performed by the liver, which carries on over thirty functions vital to life. But damage to the liver via alcohol, infection, drugs, and other less frequent causes makes the list of the top ten causes of death in this country.

The terminology of liver disease (especially chronic hepatitis) is very confusing—even to hepatologists, the superspecialists in liver disease. (Liver disease is the province of general physicians and gastroenterologists; only rarely does a physician limit his practice to the liver, and then he is legitimately called a hepatologist.) The following disease categories cover the most important points about liver disease.

Hepatitis

Since this is the most common form of liver disease (although usually not the most serious), we will begin here. The term "hepatitis" means "inflammation of the liver," which can be caused by many agents—including drugs and alcohol. But the term is generally used by the public to denote liver inflammation caused by a virus— so-called "infectious hepatitis." Viral hepatitis used to be classified as either "infectious" or "serum" because it was felt that the first type was spread primarily by contaminated clothing, dishes, etc., and the latter by needles containing contaminated blood. However, it is now known that either route of transmission can occur in both types, which are now called Hepatitis "A" and "B". Hepatitis "A" has a shorter (two to six weeks) "incubation period" (time from exposure to onset of symptoms) and is more susceptible to suppression by gamma globulin. Hepatitis "B" has a longer incubation period (six weeks to six months) and is probably not affected by routine gamma globulin. The Australian antigen (or "hepatitis-associated antigen") refers to an incomplete portion of the specific virus for hepatitis "B" which can now be identified in blood and other secretions. Of particular significance is the fact that donor blood can now be screened for this particle and rejected if it is identified, thus decreasing the incidence of hepatitis among blood recipients.

As to viral hepatitis: *Prevention* involves, first, avoiding possible sources of contamination—the oral or fecal materials (eating utensils, bedclothes, etc.) of persons with known infection; second, avoiding unsterilized needles and, third, avoiding unnecessary blood transfusions. It is impossible to completely avoid contact with hepatitis, but concern about these sources is helpful. One of the most troublesome sources in our society, of course, is the use of contaminated needles by drug addicts.

If known exposure to viral hepatitis has occurred (close contact, accidental pricking with needle used by known hepatitis victim, etc.), gamma globulin should be given to minimize the disease should it occur. Individuals traveling to an area where hepatitis is known to be a problem should receive a gamma globulin shot within two weeks of arriving and every five to six months during their stay.

Having now made the important points concerning viral hepatitis, we should point out the other three major causes of liver disease that we can do something about— drugs, toxins, and alcohol. By drugs I am now referring to ordinarily legitimate medications—such as tranquilizers and antibiotics—which can cause hypersensitivity reactions in the liver. What this means for you is that you should never take questionable medication without a doctor's direction. Toxins refer to chemicals that predictably damage the liver; an excellent example is carbon tetrachloride (often used in cleaning materials). If you work with any questionable commercial or home materials, find out if they are potentially dangerous to the liver; your physician or the state health department would be a place to start your inquiry. (Alcohol is such an important subject that I am treating it separately in this section on liver disease.

Treatment for hepatitis—whatever the cause—depends on the severity of the inflammation. Fortunately, most cases get better with conservative treatment and time. Only a very small number become rapidly severe causing death. There are chronic forms of hepatitis which require expert diagnosis and treatment; again, fortunately, these are rare compared to the large number of patients with hepatitis who return to full health.

Cirrhosis

This term is reserved for liver disease that has progressed to an advanced stage. It involves enormous medical and social problems and accounts for thousands of deaths in this country every year.

While the major cause of cirrhosis in this country is alcohol, it is important to point out that cirrhosis may be caused by many other conditions—including infectious hepatitis (though it seldom leads to this end state), drug- or toxic-induced disease, and other less well understood causes.

The treatment of cirrhosis, whatever the cause, is difficult and seldom successful in the long run. The best treatment is minimizing further damage by removal of the damaging agent—alcohol, in most cases.

Alcoholic Liver Disease

We are now ready to discuss this disease as the major cause of fatal liver disease. Some might quarrel with the description of alcoholism itself as a disease, but, in terms of its medical consequences, it is one of the deadliest diseases around. [A discussion of the social diagnostic (what is a problem drinker?), and treatment (what is the best approach to the alcoholic?) aspects of this disease is beyond the scope of this book.]

The effects of alcohol on the liver are usually described under three categories:

1. *Fatty liver:* It was taught in the past that malnutrition rather than the direct effects of alcohol (ethanol) caused this initial and completely reversible stage of liver damage. We now know that alcohol itself can directly affect the liver and that relatively small amounts of alcohol will cause temporary derangement of liver function. There is no easy way to say how much drinking is safe; truly moderate drinking does not appear to be harmful. As yet there is no evidence to suggest why some livers are more easily damaged than others, though there certainly seems to be a variation in the amount of alcohol it takes to cause problems.

2. *Alcoholic hepatitis:* This more advanced stage of liver damage requires (usually) years of heavy drinking.

While it may be reversible, it also often progresses to cirrhosis. Not all chronic heavy drinkers will develop hepatitis; women, for example, seem to be more susceptible. In one study, over eighty percent of persons with this problem had been drinking more than five years. One does not have to be consistently drunk to cause this kind of damage. Persons who recover from alcoholic hepatitis have a ten times greater chance of dying during the next three years than they otherwise would have.

3. *Alcoholic cirrhosis:* This is an end stage and irreversible form of damage. I could describe all of the possible complications of this disease, but I will simply say that most of them lead to very unpleasant endings—GI bleeding, coma, massive fluid retention, etc.

Cirrhosis is associated with a higher incidence of liver cancer. And, indeed, recent evidence suggests that alcohol intake is associated with a higher incidence of other cancers, especially when combined with smoking.

In short, alcoholism, in addition to its dire social consequences, is a devastating medical illness which affects many vital organs besides the liver—including the heart, the brain, the pancreas, and the stomach.

Ulcers

Since ulcers affect ten percent of our population, they represent a major public health problem. Ulcers are part of the folklore of this and other "advanced" societies. It has become a badge of honor and the expected in some circles. Despite such association with emotions and life-style, we still know disappointingly little about very basic causes. Hypersecretion of stomach juices, decreased tissue resistance, irritation from drugs (most commonly aspirin), and other substances (alcohol, coffee, etc.)—all seem related but none is clearly the cause. Though ulcers are usually associated with "high-strung" persons, they may occur in apparently low-key persons who avoid all possible stress. Nonetheless the avoidance of known irritants (emotional and physical) in any given case is an important preventive and therapeutic measure.

Ulcers most commonly occur in the duodenum—the first part of the small intestine just beyond the stomach—but they may occur in other areas of the GI tract. Generally they cause symptoms which are "classical"—pain on an empty stomach which is relieved by food and pain which awakens in the night. However, many ulcers produce vague symptoms, and X-ray study is still the mainstay of diagnosis. (Endoscopy—sticking a tube into the stomach—is employed in questionable cases or in cases where a direct look is important—as in ruling out cancer.)

Once an ulcer has been diagnosed, the following treatment measures must be considered:

1. *Change in life-style:* Easy to talk about but difficult to do. Sometimes in the acute phase it is necessary to hospitalize and sedate a patient in order to achieve rest and relaxation. Sometimes worry about the ulcer and the effects of illness produce a vicious cycle that is frustrating to all concerned. I have no easy answers—there usually are none.

2. *Avoidance of irritants:* This is something more realistic. Certain drugs—such as aspirin, steroids, and phenylbutazone—must be avoided if at all possible. Alcohol must be completely avoided. Smoking should

be discontinued or reduced unless severe anxiety results. Other known irritants such as caffeine (for a given individual) should be eliminated.

3. *Diet:* There are no good studies to indicate that very strict bland diets promote ulcer healing. Indeed, studies indicate that diets heavy in milk and cream lead to a higher incidence of heart attacks among ulcer victims. The best diet is one that is nutritionally sound, regular, and without known irritants.

4. *Antacids:* There is also controversy surrounding the use of antacids in terms of carefully controlled studies. However, most clinicians and patients are strong advocates of their use. When used, they must be used in amounts and intervals to do the job—which may mean hourly in early stages of healing. There are many kinds of antacids, and they are usually chosen on the basis of differing bowel effects. When used, they are best taken sixty to ninety minutes *after* a meal.

5. *Antispasmodic drugs:* There is much less agreement about the use of these drugs designed to "slow down" the GI tract. In patients with glaucoma, heart disease, and certain other GI troubles, they should be avoided. Most gastroenterologists I know don't use these drugs as frequently as antacids.

We now come to the issue of surgery for ulcers. There is no question that less ulcer surgery is being done today than thirty years ago. There are many reasons for this, but, in my mind, the major one is the availability of more nonsurgeons interested in treating ulcers. In the old days, GP's would be more inclined to turn over ulcer patients to the care of the surgeon, who would naturally be more inclined to operate. There is certainly still a role for surgery—especially for complications (bleeding, perforation, obstruction, etc.), but surgery is now considered a "last resort" rather than primary treatment. There is also some controversy as to which type of surgery is best. Unfortunately, there are no studies yet which clearly demonstrate that one type is superior to all others. The judgment of the attending medical and surgical doctors is still very important in choosing appropriate surgery.

Common GI Complaints

Finally, I would like to close this section on GI disease with a brief discussion of four common GI symptoms.

Constipation

Maybe the most succinct and inclusive description one could make of our society is that it is "bowelcentric." Some members of the human race seem more concerned about bowel regularity than any other issue in life, so let me make the point right off: There is no such thing as a "normal" bowel pattern. Once a week might be normal for some, several times a day for others. What is important is (1) not to worry about what works for you, and (2) to be concerned only about any persistent *change* from *your* normal pattern.

It is true that constipation becomes a problem as part of aging and that gentle "encouragements" (not commercial laxatives, unless needed) become useful during later years. Such encouragements (at any age) include adequate bulk intake, stewed or raw fruits and vegetables (prunes didn't get their reputation for nothing), adequate fluids, and exercise. Laxatives should be considered only a temporary help unless directed by a physician who has ruled out serious causes of persistent constipation. Some laxative preparations—especially those containing mercury—can be downright dangerous.

Having minimized this issue, I will use this opportunity to make the point that a *persistent* (more than one week) *change* in bowel habits is cause for concern; it may be an early warning sign of GI cancer and it should be investigated.

Flatulence (*Gas*)

The major cause of "gas out" is "gas in." And the major source of "gas in" (you guessed it) is air. Aerophagia (air swallowing) is very common, especially in anxiety states, and it is often unrecognized by the person involved. The second most common causes are various dietary items—milk, soda pop in large quantities, beans—or whatever else seems to do the job for a given individual.

Obviously the question of whether diagnosis and treatment is in order depends on the severity of the problem and whether the gas is associated with other, more serious symptoms. The most satisfactory approach to treatment is to eliminate the source of the gas—which means treating the anxiety underlying the air swallowing or instituting appropriate dietary modifications. Medications to "absorb the gas" or "slow down the gut" are generally far less satisfactory. One approach which may be the answer for some is "sphincter training"—learning how to better control the anal sphincter, the ring of muscle which acts as gatekeeper of the anal opening. Such "training" is a matter of the individual "holding it" (the "it" in this case being gas) with conscious effort, working up to conscious control for possible problem periods.

Halitosis (*Bad Breath*)

The point I wish to make about persistent bad breath is that there *may* be an underlying correctable cause thereby releasing you (if you so suffer) from bondage to mouthwashes. I am amazed at how many persons with this serious social problem don't know it and/or have not visited a doctor about it. Admittedly, some doctors will not get excited about this complaint, but they should. So pursue it—and include a good dentist in the pursuit. Causes of this problem can range from bad teeth or gums to lung abscesses. If nothing can be found, mouthwashes and frequent tooth brushings can indeed be helpful—but they should be a last resort.

Gastrointestinal (GI) Bleeding

Massive bleeding from the GI tract is a true emergency— as is any severe bleeding. The problem is that, since we can't see most of the GI tract, such bleeding may be occurring without signs, until the person suddenly collapses. Thus it is important to be sensitive to earlier warning signs—especially in a person who has a history of ulcer or liver disease and is therefore a higher risk for such bleeding. These warning signs include:

1. A vague but persistent and increasing feeling of lightheadedness (especially on rising) and weakness

2. Blackish stools which are foul smelling

3. Any blood from either mouth or rectum—usually via vomiting or diarrhea.

No time should be lost in getting to a hospital when GI bleeding is suspected. The death rate is significant and higher in the very young and very old. There are many studies which may be appropriate to pinpoint the cause of bleeding, and they all require the hospital. Don't waste time trying to reach your doctor and waiting for him to call back.

I again make a pitch for early diagnosis of GI cancers— especially those of the colon and rectum—by reminding you that any blood from the mouth or rectum merits investigation. Don't assume it's your hemorrhoids or the aspirin you've been taking—don't assume anything. Get it checked out.

6

Infectious Disease

This section represents a general treatise on infections. Information on specific infections is contained under the appropriate title; for example, infections of the lungs are discussed more fully under Pneumonia, those of the ear under Ear Infections, etc. But there is a basic theory that applies to all infections.

Fundamentally, there are two kinds of germs in this world, bacteria and viruses. They differ in many respects, but the difference that you must understand is this: *Bacteria usually respond to antibiotics, viruses almost never do.* It is critical that you understand this point, because far too many *unnecessary* antibiotics are prescribed in this country; not only is this an unnecessary expense, but it represents an unnecessary danger in terms of drug reactions. The vast majority of "colds" and "flu" are caused by viruses, and, considering what has just been said, these common and annoying afflictions should *not* be treated with antibiotics.

At this point you should be asking: How can I (or a

doctor) tell if my ills are caused by a bacteria or a virus? Quite frankly, the distinction is not always easy; a careful examination and some tests are required. That's one reason why doctors reach for the prescription pad—it is the easy way out. Add to this natural human tendency to "play it safe" the pressure that comes from the patient (or parents) to "do something" and you have the situation described above: unnecessary antibiotics. So back to the critical question—how to tell the difference between a viral and bacterial infection. The following are helpful in making the distinction:

1. *Patient's story:* As in any diagnostic situation, the "history" of the illness is a critical element. Location and distribution of symptoms are very important.

2. *Physical examination:* When dealing with infectious disease, the point is to search for a site of infection— i.e., a localized collection of pus (such as occurs in the tonsils) or an affected organ (such as the lungs, in which case the diagnosis could be pneumonia), or an affected system (such as the urinary). Generally, a localized infection is more likely to be bacterial, while more generalized "aches and pains" without local involvement are more likely to be viral. But there are many exceptions which have to be considered.

3. *Laboratory tests:* A CBC (complete blood count), urinalysis, chest X ray—any or all may well be indicated in a basic attempt to pinpoint or confirm infection. Many other tests involving an attempt to culture (demonstrate by growth which can be seen and identified) the offending organism are useful but take more time, usually at least twenty-four hours. In some cases, bacteria can be seen on a slide pre-

pared from various specimens (sputum, urine, etc.), but this does not represent final identification. When bacteria are not "grown" in the culture, the assumption is that a virus is the likely culprit, though the actual identification of viruses is more complex and time-consuming.

By now you should have the idea that an iron-clad distinction between viral and bacterial infection is often time-consuming and expensive. Therefore, shortcuts are sometimes taken, including the following:

1. *Prescribe antibiotics and "play it safe"*: The temptation for both patient and doctor is great. And sometimes it is justified when followup may be difficult or unlikely. But if we are going to minimize the danger of unnecessary antibiotics, both physicians and patients have to be more willing to "wait and see" when appropriate.

2. *Wait and see (watchful waiting)*: If the history, physical exam, and tests are not conclusive, if the patient is stable (even though quite miserable), and if the patient and/or family can be relied upon for followup observation, then it might be reasonable to "sit tight" and await further developments (improvement or worsening, more localization or development of clearer symptoms) before starting antibiotics. Symptoms (pain, fever, discomfort, diarrhea, etc.) can be treated in the meantime; we logically describe this as "symptomatic" versus "definite" treatment—the latter referring to treatment which attacks a known cause.

3. *Definitive treatment before final diagnosis:* Sometimes a patient is so ill that treatment with antibiotics must

be started even before final culture results are available. One of the cardinal rules of medical practice is that in such a situation antibiotics should not be started until appropriate cultures (from sputum, blood, urine, etc.) have been taken; once antibiotics are started, they tend to confuse culture results. The same rule applies to home care and is the reason why you should never take antibiotics unless so advised by a doctor.

Up to now I have been describing "typical" bugs. Unfortunately we are seeing more and more complicated infectious problems posed by unusual bugs—variants of typical strains, bugs in between bacteria and viruses in terms of the way they react to antibiotics and other characteristics. And such unusual problems require special expertise in diagnosis and treatment. Usually, a well-trained internist or family physician can handle most problems; occasionally, the superspecialist in infectious disease is required.

Given this general background, a word about the "common cold" is appropriate. The terminology for this malady is extensive and colorful: grippe, flu, "the bug," etc., are among its names. Physicians usually make a distinction between the following types of infection, based more or less on the nature and location of the complaints:

1. *URI (upper respiratory infection)*: Symptoms are well known—runny nose, watery eyes, sore throat, etc. They are confined to the "upper" structures of the breathing system—i.e., the structures above the lungs. If the infection is confined to or includes the lungs, the term pneumonia is used (see page 146). If the lungs are not involved but the infection seems to be somewhere between the throat and the lungs (as sug-

gested by a "deep cough"), the term "bronchitis" is often used to suggest that the infection is located in the trachea and bronchi—the breathing tubes leading from the throat to the lungs. By now you should have the idea that the terminology is a bit loose. The term "cold" is usually used for these symptoms when confined to the upper part of the breathing system, and it's as good a term as any.

2. *Flu:* This term is reserved for infections caused by the Influenza family of viruses. Symptoms are generally more sudden and severe—headache, high fever, total body aching, etc. Flu shots are prepared from Influenza viruses and are not effective against the common cold.

You should be prepared for the statement that most URI's and flu are caused by viruses and therefore should *not* be treated with antibiotics. This real fact is the basis for so many jokes about medical care—"take two aspirin and call me when you get pneumonia because I can treat that." The point is that viral infections, while annoying and misery-producing, will get better with time whether or not you take antibiotics. It should be obvious why people think antibiotics are great, based on their past experience of getting better while taking antibiotics; the scientific point is that they would have gotten better while swinging from a banana tree. Having belabored this, I will now go on to point out that some "colds" should be treated with antibiotics, including:

1. *Local infections:* If there is good evidence of a bacterial infection in the ears, throat, lungs, etc., antibiotics are in order. Sometimes, antibiotics will be started in suspicious cases pending final culture results.

2. *High-risk patients:* Persons who are compromised by other illnesses may be more susceptible to bacterial infections and therefore might merit antibiotic therapy. Also, the very young and the very old might be more susceptible to serious infection and therefore could be treated more readily with antibiotics.

In other words, there is still room for the exercise of the individual doctor's judgment in the treatment of "colds," but that includes the duty to consider and explain when antibiotics are not appropriate.

Several areas of controversy deserve comment. The first is vitamin C, which has been the subject of vigorous controversy within scientific circles and the subject of bemused opinion and personal testimony outside such circles. At the time of this writing—and to make a long story short—the evidence suggests that, while vitamin C does not reduce the incidence (the numbers) of colds, it *may* lessen the symptoms of a cold. The evidence for serious complications of large amounts of vitamin C is confusing. Some persons could be seriously affected and a recent report suggests that large amounts of vitamin C might destroy vitamin B-12, leading to pernicious anemia. Consultation with a doctor is in order before taking large amounts.

Now a word about "flu shots." Flu shots are prepared from past viruses that are likely to turn up again in the coming flu season for which the shots are being given. The problem is that viruses are very clever and have a way of changing themselves just enough to make the vaccine ineffective. Some exciting work is now in progress to make the vaccines more adaptable, but the final word on such vaccines is not yet in. You will, in the meantime, find some honest differences of opinion about the value of present flu shots. Most physicians agree that flu shots should be given to certain "high-risk" persons, including:

1. *The elderly:* Older citizens are generally more susceptible to bugs, including old viruses, and protection is in order.

2. *Those with chronic disease:* Any person who has another chronic (long-term) disease, and whose normal defenses might therefore be compromised, deserves flu shots. Especially included in this group are those with chronic lung disease—bronchitis, emphysema, etc.

3. *Those who are occupationally exposed:* Persons working in hospitals or clinics where the exposure rate to germs is higher may wish to have flu shots.

Now having said this, it must be pointed out that flu shots have—at best—only about a two thirds success rate. The best protection is a healthy defense system that can fight off new strains and respond well to the old germs. And I confess to never having had a flu shot yet, even though I fall into the "occupationally exposed" group. So the wisest summary advice I can give is to follow the best medical advice available to you each flu season; the actual times and numbers of shots recommended may vary from year to year.

Next a comment about cold weather, wet shoes, no hat, etc., as causes of a "cold." There is no good evidence to support any of these as a cause of the common cold. What probably happens is that cold, inclement weather forces members of the human race to crowd together indoors more often than otherwise, and the possibility of close exposure to germs is greatly increased—hence more colds.

I'm not advocating wet shoes and bare heads, but let's not overburden our kids with one more "danger warning" when they come home wet and cold and need a hug instead of a lecture.

Finally, a word about the "two aspirins and call me in the morning" advice for a cold. As indicated earlier, most "colds" will get better with time no matter what you do. But there are ways of minimizing the discomfort—and rest seems to help most anything, including colds. The pharmaceutical industry has made a fortune from cold remedies; some are worthless, others do seem to give relief for the minor aches and pains of cold miseries. In my opinion, plain aspirin, rest, and fluids are still the cheapest and best treatments in most cases.

7

cNutrition

I am not a nutritionist. But neither are many people who claim to be. That may be the most important thing I can say under the title of this section. There is an enormous amount of misinformation offered (usually for profit) by "nutritionists" without any honest credentials—which is one reason why nutrition is felt to be a "controversial" subject.

I will focus on a few subjects, again reminding you that I am not a nutritionist. I have talked with many nutritionists whom I respect because of their scientific credentials and I will share, very briefly, some of what I have learned from them.

Before I proceed to this menu of quick snacks, I would like to comment on the ethics involved in beef production by the Western world. Ronald M. Deutsch (in his book *The Family Guide to Better Food and Better Health*) describes the process in relation to the question of world needs: "As the earth's population grows, it is less and less practical to get our amino acids by the cumbersome

method of raising feed crops to support animals, then eating animals to get the crude collection of proteins they
make, and finally breaking down the proteins to get the
amino acids we wanted in the first place." I am personally
convinced that our Western wastefulness in beef production is not only an economic and health issue but a moral
issue and that we face a worldwide food crisis in part because of this wasteful chain of protein ingestion.

Calories Do Count

Good nutrition boils down to two words—*balance* and
calories. Balance implies that essential nutrients are contained in adequate (and reasonable) amounts in the diet.
Calories are contained in every food but one—water—
and they count—they add up, one after another: 3500
extra of them adds an extra pound to the body weight.

Any diet which suggests that "calories do not count" is
dead wrong. A calorie is a calorie is a calorie—no matter
where it comes from. And they all count the same, no
matter what the source. The actual definition of a calorie
is the amount of heat required to raise one kilogram
(about a quart) of water one degree centigrade. A calorie,
in other words, is a unit of heat energy. If the body does
not use up calories to provide heat energy, then they
will be stored for future use as fat and as extra weight. If
the number of calories taken in equals the number used,
the body's energy intake and expenditure are in balance
and weight will remain stable.

The equally important point is that some foods contain
more calories than others. All calories in food come from
that food's content of fats, proteins, and carbohydrates;

most foods contain some of all three. (Minerals and vitamins contain no calories.) Fat contains twice as many calories (9 calories/gram) as protein and carbohydrates (4/gram). A gram is a measure of weight, so another way of saying this is that, on a weight basis, fat contains twice as many calories as the other two major energy-containing food sources. Many people are surprised to hear that meat is as "fattening" as carbohydrates; for example, three ounces of roast beef contain more calories (270) than three slices of white bread (190). Another example: A hard-boiled egg has about the same number of calories as a boiled potato (without butter).

Calories *do* count, and the only way to lose weight is to take in fewer calories than are used up by the body. Most people are poor guessers as to the calorie content of various foods. If you are serious about losing weight and are the typical poor-guesser, you must get a list of the caloric content of various foods. (Pocket-size "Calorie Counters" are available in most drugstores.)

The belief that food eaten before bedtime will add more weight than food eaten during the day is a myth. What counts is the total energy balance over the *entire* day; it does not matter when calories are taken in or when they are used up. A piece of chocolate cake for breakfast (ugh) is just as fattening as one eaten before bedtime.

A quick word about exercise. Exercise is to be recommended for many reasons, but weight loss is not one of the greatest benefits of casual exercise. For example, to lose 200 calories (equivalent to the calories from fifty-three peanuts *or* one martini), the average person must run twelve minutes, swim thirty minutes, walk one hour, or sit in front of the television for fourteen hours. The obvious conclusion is that it would be easier to skip the peanuts or the martini. I am all for supervised exercise, but it should not be a substitute for calorie control. Also, the idea that exercise produces increased appetite is not true. Studies show that *regular* exercise is an excellent contributor to maintaining appropriate weight; it's the "quick-binge" exerciser who wants to gulp food and drink afterward.

Finally, it should be emphasized that the caloric needs of individuals can vary enormously depending on age, activity level, and pregnancy and lactation requirements. Basic metabolism (the rate at which the energy machinery of the body "runs") does decrease with age—but only about 2 percent per decade; more significant, the activity level of most people decreases with age, particularly in the decades over fifty. Pregnancy adds approximately another 40,000 calories to the energy requirements of the average woman—which breaks down to about an extra 150 calories/day (see pages 322 and 331). Women who are breast feeding require an extra 100 calories/day. But the major variable for most adults is activity level.

Balance

The word "balance" can have many definitions. In nutrition, it is usually used to imply a diet containing a wide variety of foods which can be assumed to supply the essential nutrients without significant excess of any nutrient. So, the more important word to define, nutritionally speaking, is "essential." Essential nutrients refer to those forty-seven currently known substances that must be supplied by the diet since they cannot be made by the body from other raw materials; included in this list are the famous eight essential amino acids plus such substances as vitamins, essential fatty acids, and minerals such as sodium and iron.

Since 1943, the Food and Nutrition Board of the National Research Council–National Academy of Sciences has published the famous RDA lists—lists of "recommended daily allowances." These figures are based on the best judgment of real experts—but they are judgments and not absolute certainties, and they represent "averages" and not the possible needs of a given individual. They change as new information becomes available. And they err on the side of safety by recommending more than the best estimate of what people actually need. The RDA lists should not be confused with the MDR (minimal daily requirement) lists of the Food and Drug Administration; these lists were published largely for the regulation of food products in industry and they are gradually being phased out to avoid confusion.

For the average consumer, however, "balance" still means proper amounts of fats, proteins, carbohydrates, minerals, and vitamins. These major nutrient groups are well fixed in the general public's mind and attempts to enlarge this concept are met with resistance. Nutritionists themselves still argue as to the most useful way to teach "balance" to the average housewife buying and preparing foods. In *The Family Guide to Better Food and Better Health,* Deutsch adopts the scheme of the AMA's Department of Foods and Nutrition (and its director, Dr. Philip White) and describes nine basic food groups and a way of evaluating daily diets. (Other schemes, which are based on the "basic four" or "basic seven" food groups, differ only in the categorization of foods into groups.) Whatever the method used, attention to dietary balance requires some effort, though it must be said, in all honesty, that in this country it is difficult for the person above the poverty level to avoid a reasonably well-balanced diet unless obvious faddism or strange eating habits result in diets which are limited in the variety of foods consumed.

The following summary comments should not be construed as a shortcut to thought and planning for a balanced diet. Rather, they represent an attempt to present a few basic ideas regarding some of the more important nutrient groups.

Carbohydrates

Approximately 45 percent of the calories of the typical American diet is derived from carbohydrates, including fairly simple carbohydrates such as refined table sugar and more complex carbohydrates such as the starch of cereals and vegetables. The total percentage of carbohydrates in the American diet has decreased during the past half-century; the proportion of refined sugars and syrups in the carbohydrate classification has increased remarkably; the consumption of starches has decreased. This represents a poor nutritional tradeoff, since refined sugars contain little of nutrient value other than calories, whereas foods containing starch usually contain some proteins and a variety of minerals and vitamins. Sugar also contributes to dental decay and (at current prices) to the decay of the family treasury.

Carbohydrates are an essential part of the diet, since they provide such a large amount of the energy for efficient operation of most organs and particularly the brain. If such needs are not supplied by carbohydrate foods, dietary protein or protein already existing in the body must be converted to carbohydrates in order to maintain "blood sugar" and carbohydrate metabolism at efficient levels.

Some nutritionists believe that refined (simple) carbohydrates are more likely to lead to metabolic abnormalities (such as some forms of high blood fats) than are the more complex carbohydrates of cereals, bread, vegetables, etc. It is definitely true that some forms of elevated blood fats respond to a reduction of carbohydrates in the diet.

A significant proportion of nonwhites, and a smaller number of whites, have an intolerance to lactose (the main carbohydrate of milk) due to a deficiency of an intestinal enzyme (lactase) needed to digest lactose. Such individuals may experience only mild forms of "indigestion," but it is worth thinking about in the face of "trouble with milk." On the other hand, many nonwhites have recently reduced their consumption of milk because of the wide publicity given this problem and without any evidence that they themselves have difficulty in digesting lactose. Since milk is a source of many nutrients, it should not be eliminated from the diet without sound reason.

Proteins

About 15 percent of the calories in American diets come from proteins. All protein consists of chains composed of some twenty amino acids, and dietary protein is absolutely essential because the human body cannot manufacture eight of the amino acids (nine in infants) and can get them only from outside sources of protein. Proteins are used for the purposes of both body-building and energy-providing; if adequate energy cannot be obtained from carbohydrate and fat sources, proteins are diverted to this use, thereby diminishing important building blocks for the body.

All proteins consist of these twenty amino acids used in

varying amounts and combinations. Vegetable proteins generally have fewer of the "essential" acids than found in the same amount of milk, egg, or meat protein. In order to identify these differences, proteins are often described in terms of their "biologic value." Technically this phrase describes a research determination of the amount of nitrogen from a given protein which can be used efficiently by the body. More often, the phrase is used to describe the essential amino acid content of a given protein. Some proteins are "better" than others because their amino acid content is similar to that of the proteins which the body will make from them. Egg protein has been described as the "perfect" protein, and other proteins are often measured against it to determine their relative value. (I am, for the moment, forgetting the high cholesterol content of egg yolks.) Generally, animal proteins (including the proteins of milk products) have higher biologic value than those of vegetables, although the protein of soybeans approaches the "value" of animal proteins. Vegetarians must choose their protein sources carefully to insure adequate amounts of essential amino acids. In terms of world feeding, however, plant proteins represent a much cheaper and more available source of proteins. As I have mentioned, animal protein production is generally wasteful in terms of time, labor, and plant foods required to "fatten" livestock. Actually, animal foods are more *necessary* for their vitamin B-12, vitamin D, calcium, and riboflavin than for their proteins; milk products are very adequate animal sources for these nutrients.

The quality of dietary protein is especially critical in infants. World hunger takes its greatest toll on infants; those who do not die as a result of inadequate food may have their future physical and mental abilities compromised by their inability to obtain essential amino acids during their early years. Aside from signs of obvious starvation or gross malnutrition, signs of essential amino acid deficiency are often missing until the damage has been done.

Fats

From the viewpoints of both balance and health, Americans consume too much fat. Fat should supply about 30 percent of calories; in America, fat supplies about 40 to 45 percent of the calories in the average diet. A large amount of that fat is derived from animal products such as milk fat, meat fat, and egg fat. These fats tend to be solid at room temperature, and are classed as "saturated" because their molecules hold all the hydrogen atoms they can. These saturated fats may also be a contributing factor in atherosclerosis ("hardening of the arteries"), which underlies heart disease, this nation's number one killer.

At this point, I would like to answer several commonly asked practical questions concerning fats.

1. *How can you tell which margarine is the one with the least amount of saturated fats?* If the label says "liquid" instead of "hydrogenated" or "partially hydrogenated," it should mean less saturated fats.

2. *What is the difference between "unsaturated" and "polyunsaturated" fats?* Basically, polyunsaturated means "even less saturated than unsaturated"; both are, of course, less saturated than "saturated" fats. Polyunsaturated oils tend to lower cholesterol; unsaturated oils usually neither raise or lower it.

3. *Are all vegetable oils unsaturated?* All vegetable oils *except* coconut oil are either unsaturated or polyunsaturated. Coconut oil is saturated.

Fats are important and desirable in proper amounts. They add taste to food; very low fat diets are difficult to stomach—both figuratively and literally. Two fats (arachadonic acid and linoleic acid) have been shown to be essential in infants. Dietary fats are necessary for the absorption of the fat-soluble vitamins—A,D,E, and K. But fats represent too much of a good thing for most Americans. We should all make a conscious effort to reduce the fat in our diets and particularly to reduce the saturated fats (coconut oils, solid vegetable fats, animal fats) in favor of liquid-unsaturated fats.

One of the best ways to both reduce fat intake and contribute positively to the problem of world hunger is to reduce the amount of beef, lamb, and pork in our diets. Giving up meat several days a week is something most Americans could do with a minimum of effort. Eating smaller portions of meat would have the same result. Fish and poultry (chicken, turkey) are excellent meat substitutes; they contain protein of equal biological value, generally are less expensive to buy, and have smaller amounts of saturated fat.

Vitamins

More nonsense has been perpetrated about vitamins than any other single area of nutrition. Over 300 million dollars a year are spent on vitamins; small wonder that angry opposition from manufacturers has surfaced in response to FDA proposals for regulations which would control the sale of certain vitamins.

Part of the problem is that most people do not understand that vitamins act only as catalysts; they help the body processes to work more efficiently, but are absolutely useless in and of themselves. Also, most people do not appreciate the potency of vitamins; they are very powerful in small amounts. It is really quite irrational to think that we can indiscriminately take large amounts of vitamins, which are powerful and often poorly understood in terms of long-range side effects. We would not dream of applying this "safe at any dose" thinking to other medicines or chemicals—but vitamins are often thought to be exempt from the same constraints and cautions.

It is also important to understand that vitamins are divided into two major groups, the fat soluble (which can dissolve in fat) and water soluble (which can dissolve in water) vitamins. Fat soluble (A,D,E, and K) vitamins can be stored in body fat and thus accumulate in large amounts reaching potentially dangerous levels, if taken in continual excess; water soluble (B,C) vitamins pass out in the urine and are therefore difficult to accumulate.

This is not to say that vitamins are unimportant. They are *essential* in appropriate amounts—but such amounts are rather easily obtained in the diet of most Americans. Certain groups of people are at higher risk of vitamin and other nutritional deficiencies. These groups include pregnant women; people who eat *only* restaurant ("steam table") food; people who eat the same limited variety of foods day after day for economic, health, or food-philosophy reasons; the aged, who tend to have poor eating habits; young children, whose eating habits may be abnormal; persons with bowel or malabsorption problems, etc. Such groups may indeed need nutritional guidance, including vitamin supplements. But the key word here is guidance —not haphazard devouring of large amounts of potent catalysts "just to be sure."

Having made my point, I would like to discuss three vitamins in brief form:

1. *Vitamin C:* This vitamin is discussed in the section on infectious disease and the common cold. I would again, however, like to stress that there is no evidence to support the contention that vitamin C prevents the common cold and only shaky evidence to suggest that it may lessen the effects of colds. On the other hand, there is evidence to suggest that large amounts can be dangerous (for example, kidney stone formations may result).

2. *Vitamin B-12:* Very small amounts of this vitamin are essential to the development of red blood cells. It is only found in animal food; thus "pure" vegetarians are at risk of developing B-12 deficiency. Pernicious anemia is a specific anemia (not common) which is treated with vitamin B-12 (see Anemias). Vitamin B-12 is *not* appropriate for fatigue, iron-deficiency anemias, "tired blood," or a host of other complaints. There are many unnecessary B-12 shots being given in this country.

3. *Vitamin E:* This is the latest Vitamin fad—vitamin E for everything from curing and preventing heart disease to increasing sexual performance. There is no solid scientific evidence to support *any* of these claims. Small amounts of vitamin E are necessary to normal metabolism, but increased amounts will neither cure nor prevent any diseases of mankind.

Health Foods

By now you should be able to guess what my comments will be. You're right. Most of the promotion of "health foods" is just that—promotional misinformation designed to appeal to instincts in all of us—"nature knows best," "chemicals are dangerous," etc. And make no mistake about it: The health food movement is big business for big profit, though there are many sincere advocates of the movement who are not in it for the money.

First, to put one myth to rest is to point out that all foods, to be utilized by the body, must be reduced to the simplest molecular level. At the level of molecules, the body cells cannot tell where the molecules came from—i.e., natural sources or synthetic processes.

Organic food advocates argue for more natural growing and processing—i.e., the avoidance of the fertilizers, insecticides, and additives which are essential parts of the food industry in urbanized society. The fact of the matter is that large urban populations are dependent on modern food processing for increased production and decreased spoilage of foods. Unless one literally lives off the land next to him, it is almost impossible to assure adequate and safe food without some processing. This is not to endorse irresponsible addition of chemicals to the growing or processing stages of food handling. But it is to point out that industrialized society cannot function apart from some additions to the food chain of harvest-to-mouth.

Again I rely on experts whom I respect—who say that organic foods are no better or safer nutritionally. Their only real distinction is a higher price.

Other Nutrients

I would like to list a few of the more controversial nutritional components of our diet and attempt to say what can honestly be said about them:

1. *Calcium:* There is considerable controversy among nutritionists as to the amount of calcium required by man. Milk products are the major diet source of calcium, and a diet which does not contain any milk products may carry a risk of producing health problems such as rickets in children and osteomalacia in adults. Most nutritionists agree that adults need less calcium than suggested in the past. There is good agreement that pregnant women and breast-feeding women need more calcium.

2. *Salt:* There is research evidence to suggest that continual consumption of large amounts of salt may contribute to hypertension and heart disease. Certainly people *with* these problems may have to restrict salt intake as an important part of treatment.

3. *Iron:* There is now a great controversy as to whether iron should be added to bread, as has been suggested by some nutritionists. Some nutritionists are concerned that the iron added *to* foods may not be used as effectively as the iron *in* food. Others are concerned about possible long-term danger of excess iron consumption. The final answers on this one are not yet in.

4. *Fluoride:* There is no question that appropriate amounts of fluoride in drinking water strikingly reduce tooth decay. There is no scientific evidence that fluoridated water is dangerous. (See page 271.)

5. *Lecithin:* Claims have been made that lecithin tablets will cure heart and vascular disease and make people look younger. There is no evidence to support these claims. Lecithin is plentiful in the average American diet and extra amounts will do no good.

6. *Disease cures:* Periodically, extravagant claims are made for the cure of disease—such as cancer, insanity, arthritis, etc.—by means of special diet. Aside from the well known role of dietary modification in the treatment of certain diseases (e.g., diabetes), such dietary cures are unsubstantiated.

In Summary

"We are what we eat." That statement is both obviously true and potentially misleading. We are, of course, ultimately dependent on nutritional input for the materials from which our bodies are built and with which they function. But there is a broad range of tolerance to diet variations and a remarkable adaptability to various kinds of nutrition. This is not to say that we should not all be concerned with maximally safe and effective nutrition. But it is to say that we should not be prey to the voices crying in the wilderness of ignorance and fear. Pay attention to nutrition, but do so under the guidance of those who know, from training and appropriate scientific experience, what they are talking about.

8

Women's Health Problems

At the outset I must acknowledge the difficulty I find in writing this section. There are several reasons for this. First, aside from some very basic (and important) medical problems, most of my medical activity in recent years has not included the special interests and problems of women's health. Also, I am increasingly convinced that it is difficult for a male to understand fully the unique health concerns of a woman. I fully believe that the so-called "women's liberation movement" is contributing enormously to a better understanding of modern womanhood. Finally, I am convinced that there has been a male bias in medicine. Most of this has been unintentional but nonetheless inevitable, given the dominance of males in the administration of American medicine—from selection for medical school to daily policy decisions affecting medical practice. Fortunately that is changing. I think the female viewpoint will not only provide needed change in specific areas of medical information (contraception, for example) but will add a humanizing element to American medicine that is now missing. Given the above "confessions," I will attempt to deal in this section with important health questions which are often the special concern of women, though obviously concerned males should also have an interest in such problems. Related topics in Part II include contraception, infertility, and obstetrical care.

The Role of the Gynecologist (*Obstetrician–Gynecologist*)

Previous discussions regarding the role of the primary care physician are most pertinent to this section. It is impossible to generalize on the expertise of any given primary care physician in the area of gynecology. Most primary care physicians have not kept up on the more esoteric details of female endocrinology—i.e., hormone regulation of menstrual cycles, the latest word on hormone therapy for menopause, variations in contraceptive pills, etc. For that matter, some gynecologists are not as expert in these areas as they should be.

On the other hand, most primary care physicians are fully capable of handling the two most important areas of routine female examinations—pelvics plus Pap smears and breast exams. And the capable primary care physician has the added advantage of knowing the full medical history of the woman—and not just the shape and position of her uterus.

Many gynecologists become primary care physicians to the women whose child they have delivered. Again, this practice is adequate for many basic aspects of general medicine—checking blood pressure, routine testing, etc. But the gynecologist also should know his limits and refer when appropriate.

All of which is to say that there are no "rules" as to what will work best for a given woman. As an obvious generalization, I would suggest that a gynecologist probably gives the most for the money for a woman with routine health concerns; presumably his pelvic exam is more expert (by virtue of experience) and his knowledge of hormonal-related problems more complete.

Finally, a word about women doctors for women. There is obvious rationale for this consideration, but there is also the danger that such a choice is based on the hope of being able to manipulate a "peer." For example, several female gynecologists have described to me the fairly common experience of having a female patient come to them because "you won't operate on me like those male doctors want to." I will deal with the issue of unnecessary female surgery elsewhere, but obviously the sex of the doctor should play no role in a decision as to the necessity of surgery.

The Pelvic Exam

Since I have referred several times to "a good pelvic exam," the time has come to define exactly what is meant. The following describes the elements of a routine "checkup" type exam. Obviously modifications will occur under some circumstances.

1. First, a speculum is introduced into the vagina. (This is an instrument which spreads the vaginal walls apart so that the vagina and cervix can be visually inspected and various tests can be conducted.)

2. After a thorough visual inspection, several tests can be performed. At the very least, a Pap smear of the

cervix is done. Other tests for vaginal, cervical, and urinary problems can also be accomplished at this time.

3. The final step is the so-called "internal" exam, where the examining physician inserts the fingers of one hand into the vagina while exploring against that hand with the other through the abdominal wall. The purpose of this exam is to determine the shape and location of the uterus and other pelvic structures—ovaries and tubes, etc. As a final part of this "internal," one finger is inserted into the rectum to check abnormalities of that area.

The point of this description is to give you something to measure your encounter against. If your physician—whether he is a gynecologist or other doctor—is not doing all of this as a part of your routine exams, you are being short-changed.

Surgical Treatment of the Female

There is no question that unnecessary female surgery has been done. The only question is how much, and the answer to that is almost impossible to determine. And for purposes of this discussion the more important information is how to avoid such surgery in the future.

By way of background it should be pointed out that, whereas some surgery has been deemed unnecessary in a strictly medical sense, perhaps from the standpoint of psychological improvement and preventive medicine the procedure was clearly indicated. I am not advocating such surgery, but I am suggesting that there are areas (so-called gray zones) of honest indecision which might be interpreted differently by equally competent physicians.

The classic case in point is the hysterectomy (surgical removal of the womb) in a postmenopausal woman with persistently annoying but not life-threatening bleeding. Assuming that such bleeding has not responded to hormonal treatment and/or uterine curettage, the consideration of removal to stop the bleeding becomes legitimate. It is at this point that the weighing of risks must be undertaken: the risk of surgery (though minimal) versus the risk of repeated transfusions, the risk of doing something (psychological reactions to hysterectomy do occur) versus the risk of doing nothing (the persistent annoyance and worry may eventually take their toll); the risk of overtreatment (there might be no real pathology) versus the risk of undertreatment (even though tissue studies have been normal there might be an underlying malignancy), etc. Similarly, many gynecologists prefer a vaginal hysterectomy (removal of the womb done through the vagina rather than through an abdominal incision) to tubal ligation for permanent sterilization; in the former procedure the subsequent risk of pregnancy is zero, abnormal bleeding is prevented, and, more important, cancer of the cervix and uterus cannot occur. These are examples of situations where differences of opinion frequently occur, and the surgeon might be accused of "unnecessary surgery" by a more conservative gynecologist.

So much for gray areas. What about possible black areas? Let's list a few:

1. *Bleeding problems:* Most women have abnormal bleeding (either too much or too long at the time of menstruation or in between periods) at some time in their menstrual lives. Such bleeding must always be reported to a doctor but seldom is major surgery required. What will often be required is a D&C (dilation and curettage). This is a minor surgical procedure in which the cervix (the

lower part of the uterus that protrudes into the vagina) is dilated (stretched open) to allow the scraping out (curettage) of the lining (endometrium) of the uterus (womb). This procedure is not only important diagnostically—both in determining abnormalities of the lining of the womb and in getting tissue for examination—but it often "cures" the bleeding problem and no further therapy is required.

The causes of abnormal premenopausal bleeding are many, and often a more sophisticated approach to diagnosis is required. What I am stressing here is that rarely is major surgery (such as a hysterectomy) required; this operation should be considered only after more conservative approaches have been exhausted.

Postmenopausal bleeding (bleeding which starts six months or more after the cessation of periods) is more ominous. The possibility of cervical or uterine cancer is high on the list of possibilities. Again, a D&C is the first surgical procedure (especially for diagnosis in this case), but a hysterectomy will more often be necessary since uterine cancer is a more likely cause in this age group.

2. *Fibroids:* Fibroids (also called myomas and fibromyomas) are *benign* tumors of the uterus. They are relatively uncommon during the childbearing period (ages sixteen to thirty-five), but thereafter are found quite frequently on routine pelvic examination. The point to be made here is that most do *not* require surgery. When a fibroid is first discovered, either accidentally during a routine pelvic exam or as a result of other diagnostic studies, the usual course is observation at six-month intervals. Fibroids usually disappear after the menopause since the hormonal stimulation to their growth is diminished. Some, however, will require surgical removal if they grow rapidly, cause excessive bleeding, or produce other symptoms, such as rectal and bladder pressure. The choice of the type of

surgery (total removal of the uterus or more limited procedures) will depend on many factors including the age
of the patient and the desire for subsequent child-bearing.

Again, the point of this discussion is to stress that
emergency surgery for fibroids is extremely rare and indicated only for uncontrolled bleeding or torsion (twist-
ing) of a fibroid growing on a stalk. Although the incidence of malignancy in fibroids is very small, rapid growth
in a postmenopausal woman suggests this possibility.

3. *Endometriosis:* This is a condition in which endometrial tissue (the normal lining of the uterus) grows in
abnormal locations outside the uterus, most commonly on
the ovaries. The most common symptoms are painful periods, discomfort during intercourse, and infertility. Fully
one third of infertility in the female is due to this disease.
Again the point is that seldom is extensive surgery the
first-line treatment unless the condition involves the tubes
so extensively that pregnancy cannot occur. Usually hormonal therapy will be effective in ameliorating the symptoms, and it seems to hold the disease in check. Certainly
in a woman still wishing to have children thorough conservative (nonsurgical) therapy should be attempted. Remember, however, that endometriosis is caused by
"internal menstruation" and that it is *cured* only by
menopause or ovarian removal.

4. *Surgical procedures to restore pelvic anatomy:* There
are several operations designed to correct defects in the
anatomy of the pelvic area. A brief listing of abnormalities
follows:

a. *Cystocele:* A sagging bladder which protrudes into the
vagina causing urine retention and possible infection,
or "stress incontinence" (see page 219).

b. *Rectocele:* A pushing of the rectum into the vaginal space causing constant rectal fullness and urge to bowel movement. Some women can evacuate the rectum only by finger pressure in the vagina.

c. *Uterine prolapse:* A "dropping down" of the body of the uterus into the vagina and, in extreme cases, actually protruding out of the vagina.

These conditions usually result from damage to supporting tissue during childbirth. (One of the reasons for a slow, controlled delivery is to prevent these conditions from developing in later life.) Surgery is usually the best answer for these conditions *when* they cause symptoms definitely related to the deranged anatomy. A casual finding of minor problems during routine pelvic exams in the absence of symptoms does not require surgery.

5. *Malpositioned uterus ("tipped" uterus):* This is a "problem" which sometimes exists only in the mind of the surgeon or the misinformed patient. Again, in the absence of symptoms, surgery is not required. If the malposition is secondary to an abnormality pushing the uterus out of position (such as lateral displacement by a tumor), that needs to be investigated. Most likely to cause symptoms are retroflexed ("tipped-backward") wombs. If it can be clearly established that symptoms are relieved by the use of a pessary (a device inserted in the vagina to "push" the uterus into proper position), then a more permanent cure by surgical suspension may be warranted. Often menopause with its concomitant "shrinking" of uterine tissue will take care of the problem. A "tipped" uterus does not cause infertility unless the abnormal position has been caused by endometriosis or pelvic infection; even then, it is not the malposition of the uterus which is the culprit but the disease process itself.

6. *Urinary Stress Incontinence:* This fancy phrase describes the very common situation where urine leaks during situations of increased abdominal pressure—such as laughing or coughing. It is most often caused by damage during childbirth or tissue changes after menopause. Medical treatment (including prescribed exercises) effects improvement in about half the cases and should always be tried first.

The above is a brief survey of some of the more common conditions where surgery becomes a consideration. Obviously my comments are only a guide to dealing with your physician. Ultimately, a decision becomes a matter of joint discussion between you and a doctor whom you trust.

Two final comments about surgery on the female. The first concerns a choice and the other a relatively new technique: Often there is a choice between an abdominal and vaginal hysterectomy; as mentioned earlier, the former is accomplished through an abdominal incision while the latter is done by working through the upper part of the vagina. Sometimes there is no choice—e.g., when the size or shape of the uterus precludes removing it through the vagina. But, when there is, the vaginal approach has much to recommend it *if* (and this is a large "if") the surgeon involved is skilled in that technique. The advantages are a quicker recovery period with less discomfort—nothing to sneeze at. But again I stress the experience and skill of the surgeon with this approach. Most younger gynecologists are well trained in this approach; some older surgeons prefer to stick with what they do best.

My second comment is about a new technique now being widely used, laparoscopy. This involves a very small abdominal incision (usually just below the belly button) through which a laparoscope is inserted; this is an instrument through which a good look at the "insides" is possible. This look is often coupled with the insertion of another instrument lower in the abdomen which can be used to manipulate the organs inside—or cauterize the tubes in a sterilization procedure. The great advantage of this technique is that it avoids the hazards and recovery problems of abdominal surgery; patients usually can go home within twenty-four hours. This technique finds its greatest application in diagnostic problems (where a direct look can settle the issue) and tubal ligations (sterilization of the female).

Common Complaints

I would like to comment briefly on three common female complaints. First is *vaginal discharge*. It is safe to say that every woman has this at some time or other. The causes are many, but infection is the most common. The point I wish to stress is that a *specific* diagnosis is the essential ingredient for treatment success. Too often a doctor will prescribe some kind of cream or tablets without doing a pelvic to see and test for the possible cause.

Second is *cervicitis,* a term which refers to an infection of the cervix (the lower part of the womb protruding into the vagina). The most common cause is infection associated with pregnancy. One of the most important reasons for the six-week check after delivery is to treat any cervicitis, thus preventing later problems, including a higher risk for cervical cancer. There are several legitimate methods of treatment, but cauterization in the office is very effective. Many gynecologists say that careful attention to cervicitis would greatly reduce the incidence of cervical cancer.

Third is *dyspareunia.* This large word means "painful intercourse." The causes are either emotional or physical. I mention it only to give the complaint respectability. Too many women suffer from such pain, afraid to mention it lest they be thought "strange" or "frigid." In some cases, the remedy is simple—minor surgical procedures or local medication. In other cases, particularly those related to emotional problems, the solution is more difficult but certainly worth pursuing.

Breast Cancer (*Breast Lumps*)

This is a most difficult subject to write about for many reasons. First of all, there are no shortcuts to proper understanding of this complex medical and psychological problem. Then, too, there is considerable and legitimate controversy concerning the best treatment approaches to various types and stages of breast cancer. Finally, in our breast-oriented culture, the discussion of breast cancer is inevitably clouded by understandable but often confusing emotions. Such emotions often ignore the legitimate hopes for the future and concentrates on the immediate tragedy that does all too often occur. But, in spite of these obstacles to any abbreviated discussion (as is appropriate to the philosophy of this book), I would like to attempt just that under the headings that follow.

Risk Factors

Extensive risk profiles have been developed by examining the records of patients with breast cancer. Apart from the increasing risk with age (a woman of seventy has a ten times greater risk than one of forty), most of them are too insignificant to worry about. A few, however, deserve mention:

1. *Family History:* Any woman with female relatives (especially a mother or sister) with breast cancer is at higher risk and should take advantage of early detection opportunities (see the following discussion). It should be emphasized that most women with a family history of breast cancer do *not* get breast cancer. Specifically, the risk of breast cancer in a woman whose mother or sister has had breast cancer is increased from approximately one in fifteen to one in ten— which means she still has a ten-to-one chance against developing breast cancer.

2. *Pregnancy and lactation:* The current evidence is that women who have never given birth to a full-term infant are at higher risk but that lactation (breast feeding) does not protect against breast cancer, as it was formerly thought. Women who have had their first pregnancy after age thirty-five are also in the added risk group.

3. *Hormones–birth control pills:* There is no evidence that birth control pills or hormonal treatment cause breast cancer in humans. On the other hand, there does seem to be a relationship between abnormal hormonal environments and the development of breast abnormalities, including cancer. I am deliberately vague because the evidence is not yet clear or routinely useful in diagnosing or treating breast cancer.

4. *Mammary dysplasia:* This fancy phrase refers to women who have "lumpy breasts." Again the evidence is not clear, but such women do seem to be at slightly in-

creased risk if they develop very large cysts. At the very least such women deserve closer screening and examination for the possibility of breast cancer. Since breast examination is more difficult for such women, other screening techniques (which I will mention) are particularly helpful.

5. *Breast injury:* I mention this only to say that it is *not* associated with a higher risk. Many women have discovered a breast lump when prompted to feel their breasts after an injury and have concluded a causal relationship when in fact none exists.

Early Detection
The recent Gallup survey indicates that American women still avoid the most helpful tools available for cure— monthly self-examination and immediate visits to a doctor when a questionable lump or change is discovered. I cannot honestly tell you that all breast cancer could be cured with careful early detection, but I *can* honestly tell you that *thousands* of deaths every year could be prevented with routine use of the following methods of early detection:

Monthly self-examination: This is still the mainstay of early detection; most breast lumps are discovered by accidental or intentional self-examination. For women still menstruating, six to ten days *after* the period is the best time for self-examination, since normal but confusing lumpiness is minimized. Women past the menopause often find the first day of the month easiest to remember. Teenage girls should be encouraged to start such monthly exams as a lifetime habit.

There are several ways of accomplishing adequate self-examination; the keys are being *thorough* and *systematic*. The following is a reasonable method, which can be modified as directed by your physician:

1. Start by examining your breasts in the bath or shower when they are slippery and wet. Always use the under parts (versus the tips) of the ends of your fingers. I recommend thinking of your breast as a clock and starting at the outside at each "hourly" position and working in toward the nipple. Another method is to circle the breast, starting at the outside and working in decreasing circles toward the nipple. However you cover the breast, you should gently press the breast tissue against the underlying ribcage (chest wall) to feel any unusual masses or lumps.

2. After drying off, visually examine your breasts in front of a mirror, looking for any obvious change in shape, skin texture, nipple position, etc. This visual exam should be done both with arms at your side and with both arms folded overhead. (When the arm is held overhead, the muscles under the breast are put on a stretch and the breast tissue is distributed in a manner more suitable for both manual and visual examination.)

3. Reexamine your breasts as you did in the shower while sitting on the edge of your bed. Examine each breast visually in front of a mirror (with the opposite hand) both with the arm down and overhead.

4. Finally, and probably most important, examine each breast again while lying down. Examine, as above, with the opposite hand, both with the arm along the side and above the head. Putting a pillow or towel behind the shoulder of the side to be examined is often useful in distributing the breast tissue more evenly over the chest wall, thus making examination easier.

Again I stress that the actual method is probably less

important than the fact that you do it *thoroughly* (in the various positions described), *systematically* (in a way that covers the entire breast), and *monthly*. Every breast is different and each woman learns to know the normal state of her breasts if she is regular in self-examination. Indeed, a woman who practices careful monthly examination becomes more skilled at detecting change than the physician who may examine only yearly.

Physician examination: As just suggested, a yearly breast examination by a physician or other trained person is no substitute for monthly self-examination. However, the yearly exam is important and should be insisted upon as part of any physical examination in a woman over eighteen. You're getting gypped if you don't get a breast exam as part of any physical exam.

Mammography: Mammography is a special X-ray technique which provides a much better "look" at the soft tissue of the breast than does routine X ray. Special machines and film are involved and experience at interpretation is required. Done properly, mammography offers a tremendous assist in both early detection (screening) and interpretation of lumps found on examination. Like regular X ray, it is a quick and painless procedure.

Most authorities now recommend yearly mammography (over age thirty-five) when appropriate equipment which minimizes radiation exposure is available. More frequent examination may be required in a high-risk female or one with previous breast disease. If yearly mammography examination is not possible, it should be arranged as often as possible and certainly no less than every three years.

Thermography: This technique, which uses a special heat sensor to pick up heat waves, has proven useful as a screening technique; it does not involve radiation. When abnormalities are detected, they must be investigated further with examination and mammography. While thermography is a valuable tool, it is not at present as widely available as mammography. Good early detection can be practiced by the use of examination and mammography, and the unavailability of thermography should not discourage active early detection programs.

Diagnosis and Treatment

Now we come down to the nitty-gritty. What should be done when a lump or other suspicious abnormality (change in skin, nipple discharge, etc.) is discovered? First, remember that about eighty percent of all lumps turn out to be something other than cancer; those are fairly decent odds and should encourage a positive approach. Second, seek the immediate evaluation of a primary physician, gynecologist, or general surgeon as soon as possible; time may be of the essence and even a week's delay could be damaging.

We now face squarely the question of "what kind" of doctor to go to initially. Most primary care physicians—internists, gynecologists, family doctors—will send breast problems to the general surgeon, who has the total experience of evaluating the lump, doing the biopsy, and performing the surgery when necessary. Some gynecologists trained in general surgery will also do such total care but most will refer to the general surgeon. So going to the general surgeon right off will often save time and money.

Once a lump has been discovered, actual diagnosis by the general surgeon is the next step. Generally, one of three courses will be recommended:

Wait and see: Some lumps are so unlikely to be cancer and so likely instead to be related to hormonal changes of the menstrual cycle that the surgeon will advise careful observation over several weeks to see if the lump does not regress and/or disappear. Admittedly this wait may be anxiety-producing, but it does have the merit of avoiding surgical biopsy. If, after several weeks, the issue has not been settled, biopsy should be performed. (Biopsy here refers to removal of some of the suspicious tissue for examination under the microscope.)

Biopsy outside the operating room: In some cases, a biopsy for absolute certainty will be performed in the office or minor surgery department. Sometimes using a needle to obtain tissue for study rather than cutting the tissue out will be appropriate. The more common biopsy is removal (under local anesthesia if done outside the operating room) of the questionable lump for examination under the microscope; such removal generally does not affect the appearance of the breast, except for a very minor scar.

Biopsy in the operating room in preparation for possible surgery: When there is any reasonable suspicion of cancer, this is the course that is most commonly recommended. The idea is to avoid two surgical and anesthetic exposures. If the biopsy specimen as examined by frozen section clearly shows cancer, then the surgeon can proceed immediately with the necessary surgery; fortunately, frozen section examination of breast tissue is highly accurate and usually allows such immediate decision. Obviously all the alternatives must be thoroughly discussed before entering the operating room. Some women prefer a two-stage process with time after the biopsy to talk and think; others prefer making all the possibly necessary decisions beforehand, thus allowing a single operative procedure.

We have now come to the most critical question of all in this discussion. What *is* the best treatment for breast cancer? Do more localized operations ("lumpectomies") offer the same chance of cure as more traditional "radical" operations—which also remove associated lymph nodes and underlying muscles? Is radiation as effective as surgery? Obviously these are terribly crucial questions because of the psychological impact of breast surgery in our society. Unfortunately the only totally honest answer that *anyone* can give to these and similar questions is that we do *not* have clear and satisfactory answers.

In September 1974 (only a few days after surgery had been performed on Mrs. Betty Ford), preliminary results were released from the National Cancer Institute study of breast disease. (This study, under the direction of Dr. Bernard Fisher of Pittsburgh, is a cooperative effort of over thirty medical centers to answer questions concerning breast cancer treatment.) Many people were misled by news reports stating that this study has proven that radical surgery is not necessary. As Dr. Fisher was careful to point out, the data released at that time (September 1974) was very preliminary and based on only two years of followup. Meaningful data on treatment of breast cancer requires at least five years (preferably ten) of followup. Previous studies have suggested prematurely that other treatment forms were as effective as radical surgery only to change recommendations later when longer followup data became available.

Until studies provide firm answers, I want to state my own opinion. (I remind you at this point that I am not a surgeon and that I am extremely sensitive to unnecessary surgery. This opinion is based both on personal examination of the data available and on extensive discussion with many physicians, both surgeons and nonsurgeons.) To begin with, I believe that radical surgery—meaning surgery which involves removal of the entire breast plus at least associated lymph nodes—still offers the best chance of permanent cure in carefully selected instances of cancer where the disease still appears to be localized to the breast in question. The reason for this is that microscopic bits of cancer are often found in the tissue and nodes removed by radical surgery; such tissue would have been left behind if less radical surgery had been performed. This is not to say that less radical procedures cannot remove all the cancer and therefore be curative, but at present we cannot tell when such procedures will work. Like any human being, I would like to see other less mutilating forms of treatment proven as effective in eliminating such cancer, but as yet that proof is lacking and it would be dishonest to suggest otherwise. It is terribly unfortunate that comparative studies were not done years ago when radical surgery was first introduced, but we are now left with a procedure which has proven effective in properly selected cases and we must await belated proof that other forms of therapy are as effective.

A second point: There are cases when radical surgery is performed when it should not be—as in advanced cases where there is little chance of cure and other palliative procedures would be just as effective and less mutilating. There is no easy way to avoid this kind of ill-advised surgery, except to be aggressive in questioning the surgeon with whom you are dealing. Specifically, you should be prepared to ask about proposed treatment in a manner that suggests you wish to participate in the decision but are open to the evidence presented. This is one of those times when it is appropriate to ask the physician what would be recommended if it were "a member of your family."

Beyond these general statements, it would be dangerous for me to be more specific. Each case must be individualized, both medically and psychologically. The age of surgery by dictum is and should be over. You have every right to be a part of the decision process, and, if your surgeon is reluctant to share his thinking with you, find another.

Postsurgery

When and if surgery is performed, a perfectly normal life is possible, though at times that goal will seem distant. The Reach to Recovery program of the American Cancer Society has made us aware of the benefits of emotional and physical support in the period following breast surgery. If your doctor does not suggest such support, ask about it. Don't be afraid to share doubts and ask apparently stupid questions. Generally, you will find more help than you could have hoped for, but sometimes it takes asking to bring it.

In Summary

Breast cancer is, legitimately, a frightening disease—but it can and should be less so. Most women do *not* get breast cancer. Early detection can pay off. Permanent cures do occur by the thousands every year. People do survive breast surgery to lead normal lives. The keys to a positive approach are:

1. Immediate consultation with a competent and understanding general surgeon when a lump is discovered.

2. Consultation with Reach to Recovery (American Cancer Society) or similar resources when surgery becomes necessary.

3. Unashamed use of spiritual and emotional support resources—clergymen, family, etc. This is no time to be ashamed of fear or ignorance. I have found that professional and nonprofessional people are almost always ready to lend a hand with the emotional needs of the victims of this disease, but they must sometimes be alerted to those needs that are not apparent.

Uterine and Cervical Cancer

I have put these two cancers of the female reproductive tract together for several reasons. First, they are often confused in terms of diagnosis and treatment. Second, they are both eminently curable if diagnosed early. And, third, they are the most common cancers of the female after breast and colon cancers.

A quick lesson in anatomy is in order. The uterus (or womb) is a pear-sized and -shaped organ (except during pregnancy) which is located deep in the pelvis. The lower part of the uterus is called the cervix, and it alone projects into the vagina and is therefore accessible to direct visualization during routine pelvic examination. Thus only the cervix can be seen and scraped by the Pap smear method, and only cervical cancer can be reliably screened by the Pap smear. Screening and diagnosis of uterine cancer (which is a cancer of the inner lining called the endometrium) can be accurately accomplished only by a D&C—a procedure wherein the cervix is dilated (the "D" of D&C) so that an instrument can be inserted to curettage (scrape) out the inner layer of the uterus (the "C" of D&C). Newer methods of suction curettage are now available as in-office procedures.

Having made this important distinction in diagnosis between these two cancers, a further description of each is in order according to the following categories.

Cause and Risk

The cause of these two common cancers is unknown. However, it is clear that *cervical* cancer is related to irritations of exposure (remember that it projects into the vagina), and the most common exposure is sexual intercourse. Thus, cervical cancer is more common in women who have extensive, early, and varied sexual intercourse (with many partners). The actual irritant (or irritants) involved is not clear, but there is increasing evidence that a virus of the herpes family may be involved. Sexual intercourse is not a contributing factor in *uterine* cancer, though infertility and lack of regular ovulation are associated with it.

Screening and Diagnosis

Since both cancers are slow growing and very curable in early stages, the emphasis must be placed on screening. Cervical cancer, for example, takes about ten years to reach the invasive stage of penetration into deeper tissues; the time of such invasion is less in uterine cancer, but it is also slow.

As emphasized above, the Pap smear is the screening method for *cervical* cancer. It is very reliable when done properly. (Other methods of self-scraping or self-rinsing to obtain cervical cells for examination are as yet not as reliable as the traditional Pap smear scraping performed by a physician or other appropriately trained person.) Since cervical cancers "in situ" (noninvasive) are theoretically 100 percent curable, and since Pap smears are designed to detect such cancers, and since it takes about ten years for cervical cancers in situ to become invasive, deaths from cervical cancer are preventable. Yet thousands of women die from this disease every year in this country. While some of these deaths stem from errors of diagnosis and treatment, the vast majority are due to women not having yearly Pap smears from age twenty-one on. Surveys indicate that over half the women in this country have never had a Pap smear. (Since Pap smears are so often misunderstood, I have a special section on them later on.)

There are other methods of screening for cervical cancer, but they are much more specialized and therefore less available. Techniques such as colposcopy are used more in confirmatory diagnosis than is mass screening.

It is more difficult to screen for *uterine* cancer. Office suction curettage or endometrial biopsy may detect this cancer, but if it is small it may be missed. Therefore, a D&C is the ultimate diagnostic procedure. Since this is a much more extensive procedure than the Pap smear, it is not done routinely as a screening test for uterine cancer. The Pap smear picks up abnormal cells from the uterine lining in about fifty to sixty percent of patients with uterine cancer.

What about symptoms—particularly of uterine cancer, since no simple screening test exists? Unfortunately, early cancers in both the cervix and uterus can exist without any symptoms. But there are warnings which must be investigated. They include bleeding, which is often passed off as "my uterus kicking up" or "one last fling at menstruation." *Any* postmenopausal bleeding is highly suspicious of uterine cancer.

At this point it is important to emphasize the difference between screening and diagnosis. Screening is based on examination of cells that have been scraped or collected in fluid. Diagnosis is based on microscopic examination of tissue. In the case of uterine cancer, the D&C provides the necessary tissue. But, in the case of cervical cancer, the Pap smear does not. Any diagnosis of cervical cancer (and consequent treatment) requires a biopsy specimen which can be obtained from the cervix in several ways.

The Pap Smear
The Pap smear should be done at least once a year in women over twenty-one (and more often in certain high-risk groups such as those who have had previous abnormal smears). It is a simple and painless procedure which can and should be done as a part of every annual pelvic examination. It involves gently scraping cells from the cervix and placing them on a slide for examination under the microscope.

Pap smears are reported in various *classes* (1–5). (These classes are not to be confused with clinical *staging* or the extent of invasive cancer.) Class 1 indicates all normal cells. Class 2 ("atypical benign") smears are seen in patients with infections such as monilia, trichomoniasis, or cervicitis. Class 3 smears may be due to severe infection but are more commonly associated with a premalignant phase known as "dysplasia"; such smears must be repeated immediately and the cervix should be biopsied to obtain an accurate tissue diagnosis. Class 4 smears are usually found when the cervix contains areas of "carcinoma in situ"—a later stage of dysplasia; again, biopsy or "conization" should be done. Class 5 smears are characteristic of invasive cancer.

Again I emphasize that a Pap smear does not constitute diagnosis. Even a class 5 smear must not be accepted as basis for treatment until a biopsy has been done.

Treatment

The treatment for noninvasive (in situ) cancers of either the cervix or uterus is surgical removal of the entire uterus and cervix; in the case of uterine (endometrial) cancer, the tubes and ovaries are always removed. However, in young women with in situ endometrial cancer, reversion of the process has been produced by administration of potent progesterone-type hormones. If the cancer of either is invasive, then treatment becomes much more complex and individualized, involving radiation and possible further surgery.

One exception to the above is cervical cancer in situ in a young woman who wishes to have children. In such cases, sometimes a wide excision of a cone-shaped portion of the cervix is done, leaving the uterus. Such a procedure involves a definite risk and such a woman must be followed very carefully with Pap smears and other examination to make sure no cancer is left or is recurring.

One common question is whether a woman who has

had her uterus removed (including the cervix) needs to have Pap smears. It the uterus was removed because of cervical, uterine, or ovarian cancer, Pap smears should be done to rule out recurrences in the remaining vaginal wall. If the uterus was removed for conditions other than malignancy, a Pap smear probably does not need to be done. However, for absolute safety it won't hurt, and since pelvic exams should continue on a yearly basis even after removal of the uterus it is simple enough to do the Pap smear at the same time.

Menopause

Menopause is defined as the absence of menstrual periods for one year. The natural development of this final cessation usually occurs over a period of several years, marked by increasing irregularity. In this country, about thirty percent of women will experience menopause by age forty-five; by age sixty, 100 percent will. Since menstruation depends on normal ovarian hormones, anything that interferes with ovarian function can produce cessation of menstruation before the natural occurrence; surgery involving removal of the ovaries is the most common cause of such "premature" menopause.

Many physicians are now adopting the view that menopause represents a hormone-deficient status (like diabetes) which should therefore be treated with hormone replacement. While this may be somewhat oversimplified, since many women do not become estrogen deficient until their very late years, it does represent a more legitimate approach than the view which writes off middle-age problems as "psychological." While there may indeed by a psychological component to the problems of middle age in both men and women, it is the obligation of the physician to search for organic causes of symptoms afflicting the middle-aged woman—and not just superficially pass them off as "that time of life."

On the other hand, superficial views suggesting that estrogens are the answer to all female problems of life are also misleading. There is no evidence to promise that estrogens given before menopause will delay the aging process, that estrogens given after menopause will restore youth, or that outside sources of estrogens will prevent atherosclerosis (hardening of the arteries) or osteoporosis (thinning of bones). (Notice: I am not talking about the unquestioned protective effect of the female's own hormones in protecting against "hardening of the arteries" and "thinning of bones." What I am saying is that extra hormones given before or after menopause do not offer this protection.) All that can be said with certainty is that, where true estrogen deficiency exists and there are symptoms clearly related to such deficiency (hot flashes, insomnia, and a thinned-out vaginal lining causing painful intercourse and itching), estrogen replacement therapy will have a high probability of correcting these specific problems. A vaginal smear (cells gently scraped from the lining of the vagina) will easily demonstrate the level of estrogen; if it is low and there are symptoms, it is quite rational to treat such symptoms with preparations of estrogen.

Once it has been determined that symptoms attributable to estrogen deficiency exist, the question arises as to what kind and amount of hormone to give. Three of the common questions asked are as follows:

Is natural estrogen (Premarin) better than synthetic estrogens? There is no evidence to suggest greater superiority or safety for the natural hormone preparation. Some women find the natural hormone more tolerable in terms of side-effects (particularly nausea).

Do such hormones cause cancer? There is no statistically significant evidence to support this contention.

Should androgens and/or progesterones also be taken in menopause? Except in specialized situations, there is no controlled, double-blind evidence to prove that such hormones are useful in routine menopausal hormone replacement.

The question as to what kind of physician is best able to handle the problems of menopause is a difficult one to answer. Certainly the gynecologist is best equipped to handle the strictly hormonal and pelvic problems associated with the middle years of the female; any complicated problems in these areas should be referred to a gynecologist. On the other hand, a good primary care physician who can also handle the other medical—and psychological—problems of the middle-aged woman (who, after all, is more than just a specimen of estrogen deficiency) has much to be recommended, if that physician also has a reasonable grasp of specific estrogen-deficiency problems. There is no rule on this one; each individual has to choose on the basis of what is available. I am simply making, again, the point that middle-aged life and health are more than just giving estrogen.

One word of warning is crucial: Any bleeding occurring after menopause has been established should be investigated immediately. In a significant number of such cases (up to one third) such bleeding is a sign of cancer of the uterus. A "D&C" is required for the diagnosis of such cancer; a Pap smear is reliable only for the screening of cervical cancer and does not reliably pick up cancer cells from the lining of the uterus.

It is *extremely* rare for a woman to become pregnant

after one year of no periods. But until then, birth control should be used. Children born of pregnancies occurring after the mother is forty have a one-in-seven chance of mongolism; amniocentesis should be strongly considered in any pregnancy past that age.

Masters and Johnson have highlighted the possibility of an active sex life past the age of menopause; their research points out that couples with an active sexual life can expect to continue such a relationship into their sixties and seventies. Intercourse that is painful for the female due to thinned out vaginal tissue will often respond to estrogen therapy and vaginal lubricants.

Finally, many psychologists are telling us that a life-style that is healthy before menopause is likely to be so during the middle years—and vice versa.

A Dictionary of Other Health Problems

Acupuncture

It would be impossible for me to ignore this subject—it is a "happening" both medically and socially. I am personally convinced that acupuncture will find a useful but limited role in Western medicine as it obviously already has in Oriental practice.

Most observers of acupuncture feel that its primary role will be in the relief of pain. Contrary to popular belief, acupuncture is not widely used in China for surgical anesthesia; it is used in less than one percent of all operations in China and then often in conjunction with other, more traditional forms of anesthesia and pain relief. Nor is there any solid evidence that it cures disease of an organic (that is, with real tissue damage) nature.

Acupuncture is now being widely investigated according to the same rigorous techniques of double-blind investigation that we demand of other new treatment forms. (Some argue that we should simply accept the "results" of long-term use in other societies as evidence of its effectiveness.)

Some have interpreted the caution of established medicine in this country as typical conservatism or reactionary politics. I would not deny this element of American medicine, but in this case I think caution is entirely justified; it represents the same careful evaluation we should expect and demand for any new drug or treatment before it is approved for general use.

There is already evidence to warrant further investigation as to the appropriate role and use of acupuncture. My great concern is that understandable public pressure from those for whom traditional medical knowledge can provide no further treatment will short-circuit careful investigation and control of this new tool. There are many reports of complications, of missed and treatable conditions, and of outrageous charges stemming from acupuncture performed in less than ideal settings. Until we know more about the appropriate role of acupuncture and until its practice is more carefully controlled, the "buyer must beware." I'm not saying flatly to avoid it—but be careful of your body and your pocketbook. And be very suspicious of acupuncture performed as a promise to cure disease rather than treat symptoms. Insist that a careful diagnosis be established as part of the process; don't seek acupuncture as a blind treatment for symptom relief.

Allergy Problems

The terminology of the allergy field is confusing to both physicians and the public. New discoveries and rearrangement of old experience change the lingo almost daily. But, for our purposes, there are two basic kinds of problems to know about—those allergic reactions that occur suddenly and are potentially life threatening and those which are more chronic.

Reactions

Life-threatening allergic reactions can arise in one of two ways. Most fearsome are those reactions that arise in response to some "stimulus" (technically called an antigen), such as venom from an insect bite, drug reactions (penicillin is the most common, in part because it is used so much), food reactions, etc.; in severest form such reactions lead to difficulty in breathing and collapse of the cardiovascular system (so-called "anaphylactic shock"). Such reactions usually occur soon after the stimulus but may delay for hours or weeks. Immediate treatment is mandatory; no time should be wasted in seeking emergency care at the nearest medical facility. Persons who have had such reactions should: (1) take great care to avoid such stimuli in the future; (2) arrange to carry emergency treatment kits when emergency care will not be readily available; (3) arrange to carry Medic-Alert (or similar) identification alerting medical personnel to such allergy problems. The other way in which life-threatening problems arise is through the exacerbation (a fancy word often used in medicine to describe a condition or disease as it gets worse) of a known allergy problem, such as asthma. Usually this process is more gradual and there is more time to seek help.

Another category of allergic reactions should be mentioned at this point—namely, those annoying, sometimes frightening skin reactions that occur, often rapidly, in reaction to many causes—virus infections, drugs, or unknown stimuli. Such rashes may vary from little red spots all over to big, frightening welts (hives, or urticaria). They usually itch. Fortunately they usually can be easily controlled with injectible and oral medications (antihistamines are usually sufficient), and they usually do not recur with any degree of regularity.

Most people with allergy problems are harassed by the more chronic—though often terribly annoying—symptoms of "allergic rhinitis" (including hay fever) that we all know about: wheezing, runny nose, weepy eyes, nasal drip. However, these allergy problems pose real problems of choice for the individual so afflicted. Those choices revolve about the following questions:

1. Are my symptoms due to an allergy—and, if so, what am I allergic to?

2. What kind of doctor should I go to?

3. Can "allergy treatments" really help me?

I should tell you, right off, that the answers to the above questions are not usually clear or easy—that's the problem faced by the medical consumer. Many of the symptoms which can suggest allergy can also be caused by other medical problems (viral infections, chronic sinusitis, etc.). Often it is impossible—even after extensive skin testing—to identify the cause of allergic symptoms. And, quite frankly, some doctors who call themselves allergists have not had formal training and/or are in the business for the quick money and the good hours. Finally, while allergy treatments can offer dramatic help for some sufferers, for many others treatment will make little difference except in the size of your pocketbook.

So what's a sufferer to do? First and foremost, this is one of those medical situations where reliable advice from an objective medical source is most crucial. If you have a good relationship with a primary care physician or facility, start with that. *Don't* go directly to an allergist just because you think you have an allergy. Some primary care physicians are competent to handle allergy problems; at the very least, they can advise you as to further care. If money is no problem, you have little to lose besides time and effort by going to a recommended allergist. But if money comes hard, as it does to most, I would go to an allergist with some very specific questions in mind:

1. Do you think you can give me some very specific help?

2. What are the chances of the time and money I spend with you "paying off?"

I'm not saying that anyone can give full answers to the above, but by asking such questions you will put the doctor in a position of knowing that you are concerned about cost and results and that you expect a reasonable accounting of what's going on. Such questions may incline an allergist to follow a more reasonable approach to your problem than he might otherwise take.

All of this is not meant to diminish the real help competent allergists can offer some people. But it is to say clearly that allergy is a field where the "buyer must beware." Advice from a knowledgeable and objective third party should be diligently sought before going to just any doctor (or clinic) that advertises expertise in allergies.

Anemias

An anemia represents a condition in which the quality and/or quantity of blood is less than it should be. Maybe a better definition for our purposes is blood which is not able to perform as it should—carrying oxygen by means of red blood cells to the body tissues. In that sense, the lay and advertising phrase "tired blood" has some meaning, though it can also be very misleading if it suggests that "pep pills" or "tonics" are the answer. The vast majority of fatigue is *not* due to an anemia or any kind of "tired blood." It is more often due to tired spirits and tired bodies and should be approached at that level.

The most important point I can make about anemias is that there are many different kinds of anemia, each with its own specific treatment. In order to treat an anemia effectively, an accurate diagnosis must be established. And in order to establish an accurate diagnosis, a careful study of the blood, often requiring several tests, must be done. A simple hematocrit or hemoglobin determination is *not* enough to establish the type of anemia initially; once a diagnosis has been made, such simple determinations may be useful in following the progress of treatment.

The second most important statement I can make is that, along with a diagnosis as to the type of anemia, it is important to establish the cause of a given anemia. What I am really saying is that many anemias are caused by blood loss that may not be obvious unless searched for. And such internal blood loss may be an early warning sign of cancer. So this question should always be asked in the face of a newly discovered anemia: What is causing it? *You* should ask the question when the diagnosis is made.

An accurate diagnosis must be made as to type and cause—only then can appropriate treatment be instituted. It is true that most anemias turn out to be iron-deficiency anemias without serious cause which can be treated with iron supplement medication. But *many* anemias are not that simple. They need entirely different kinds of treatment, and equally important, they may signal serious disease—silent ulcers, silent cancers, etc.

A good primary care physician is usually sufficient to make the initial diagnosis and start treatment. In complicated cases, the skills of a hematologist (a subspecialist of internal medicine) will be useful.

But, again, neither you or your doctor should ever assume "tired blood" and start iron tablets without careful diagnosis. The diagnosis of iron-deficiency anemia, for example, requires a full blood count (with careful attention to the smear) and determination of indices, total iron, and iron-binding capacity—as a minimum. And, in most cases, particularly in males (where menstrual bleeding would not be a likely cause), a thorough search should be made to find the reason for an iron-deficiency anemia.

Arthritis

The most important point to be made about joint pains is this: Most joint pains are *not* due to rheumatoid arthritis but to one of over 100 recognized causes of joint pain, many of which are completely curable. The second most important point is this: Even if joint pains are due to rheumatoid arthritis, arthritis is a disease which can be controlled or cured in the majority of cases.

Most people have the idea that all joint pain is due to arthritis and that since arthritis is untreatable it isn't important to see a doctor about joint pains. Considering what I've just said, that's obviously not true. Now, I'm not suggesting that you get every little joint twinge checked out; there are not enough doctors around to do that. But any persistent and severe joint pain that makes you take pain medicines and/or limits your activity merits investigation.

The big question at this point is what kind of doctor to go to. If you have a satisfactory relationship with a primary care physician I would begin there. Quite frankly, however, chronic joint disease is the kind of problem some doctors aren't too interested in. So if you're not getting satisfaction I would not hesitate to see a rheumatologist— a doctor who specializes in joint diseases. Now I also have to warn you that such doctors usually make extensive investigations and are therefore expensive. Their studies may include X rays, blood tests, removal of fluid from joints for study, etc. But, if you have a severe problem with one or more joints, it is money well spent (within reason).

Rheumatoid arthritis—the most feared form of joint disease—is a disease that should be treated vigorously and early. Unfortunately most patients and many doctors give up too easily. There are some rheumatologists who insist that every patient with a definite case of *rheumatoid* arthritis should be tried on gold (or less often chloroquine) therapy because these drugs seem to be the only ones which can actually arrest the disease; many others can be used to alleviate the symptoms. In addition to drugs, much can be done using heat, physical therapy, etc. But both patient and doctor must work at it!

Also to be considered are surgical procedures on affected joints, including joint replacements. Indeed, one of the great developments in medicine in the past twenty years has been the development of "total hip replacement" surgery. As the name suggests, the operation involves removing the damaged joint and replacing it with a joint composed of synthetic materials. To be more specific, the damaged upper end of the thighbone is removed and replaced by a metal piece inserted into the remaining thighbone. Then the damaged area of the pelvic bone is cleaned out and replaced by a plastic cup into which the new metal upper of the thighbone inserts. Presto—a new joint! (Incidentally, one of the most difficult parts of developing this surgery was to find a safe and effective "cement" to hold these new parts in place; the substance currently being used—methacrylate—is a plastic used commercially under the name of Lucite.)

Obviously I have oversimplified the procedure and minimized the risks involved. Before listing some of the "qualifications," however, I want to indicate clearly that this operation is so effective for severely damaged hip joints that other operations formerly used are no longer worth talking about. Total hip replacement is dramatically effective in ninety percent of cases; about five percent will suffer from some complication of the surgery and another five percent will not demonstrate the usual improvement. Also, the following contraindications—reasons for not doing the surgery—should be considered:

1. Generally, persons under age fifty are not eligible for the surgery. This limitation stems from the fact that experience with current materials extends back only about twelve years, and doctors are still not sure how wear and tear will affect longrange results. Having said this, many exceptions to the "age fifty" rule are made for truly severe disability.

2. Persons with a current or past history of infection in the hip area are not generally eligible for surgery. In the past, infection was an absolute contraindication —no exceptions. Today, several centers are experimenting with operations on individuals with infection; preliminary results are encouraging.

3. Persons with less than severe pain or disability are not operated on. Quite often a person who is able to function, but not as well as he would like, requests this operation in order to "get back to normal." First, it should be stressed that this operation will not restore function

to complete normalcy. It will dramatically improve pain—virtually eliminate it, in fact—and also improve function; but a person will not be able to do things which put sudden stress on the joint (jumping, bouncing, etc.). Second, it must always be remembered that the surgery is "major" and not without significant, though minimal, risk. As with everything in medicine, risks must be weighed. The improvement of minimal disability is not worth the risk involved.

One of the side benefits of the development of this operation has been the investigation of other joint replacements. Currently, knee replacements are being done; the results are somewhat less satisfactory and the length of followup experience less than with hip replacements. Ankle, elbow, and shoulder replacements are being done experimentally; they are not available routinely. Joint replacements in the hand are done widely and with excellent results.

Finally, a quick word about "fad" or "quack" cures for arthritis. Rheumatoid arthritis is one of those diseases that is marked by a natural up-and-down course; in other words, without doing anything many patients get better. Thus it is a natural for special remedies—copper bracelets and the like. My own attitude is this: As long as the proposed cure does no harm (except to your pocketbook) and as long as you seek expert advice and care, why worry about a copper bracelet or two? What does concern me greatly, however, are those who substitute these "cures" for the expertise that is available.

I'd like to summarize what I've been trying to say: First, there are over 100 causes of joint pain. Don't assume it's rheumatoid arthritis until you have seen a doctor competent to make the diagnosis—and this requires more than just a quick examination. Many forms of joint pain are curable, so it's important to find out exactly what the problem is. Second, if it turns out to be rheumatoid arthritis, don't give up. The vast majority of sufferers can be successfully treated and helped; the cases of crippling we are all familiar with are a small minority—and many of those would have benefited from drugs and surgery earlier in the disease.

Asthma

Asthma is often divided into "extrinsic" and "intrinsic" forms. The former represents asthma triggered by some outside, allergic stimulus such as pollen or animal hair; the latter is triggered by some nonallergic stimulus, including emotional upset, change in humidity or temperature, etc. Both forms result in the typical syndrome of frightening "air hunger" and wheezing caused by excessive secretions and muscle contractions in the air tubes of the lungs.

The treatment of the acute asthma attack is fairly well standardized; fortunately, most acute attacks can be aborted rather easily with appropriate medication. The more difficult and challenging task is to prevent such attacks from occurring in the first place. The following information is pertinent to that task:

1. If attacks are severe and frequent, a search for the offending allergic causes is worthwhile; make an appointment with a good allergist.

2. Most physicians who take care of asthma patients are impressed with the role of emotional upset in triggering attacks. Attention to this factor can be very worthwhile.

3. A new drug, cromolyn, has been recently introduced in this country for use in *preventing* acute attacks; it has no role in the *treatment* of acute attacks. Long used in England, the drug appears to be effective and safe in appropriately selected patients.

I would close by emphasizing the emotional component in this disease. Attention to this by all concerned—physician, family, patient—should be fundamental to any treatment program.

Back Pain

"My aching back" is both a symbolic complaint and a real physical problem for millions of people; it is not surprising that these words have been adopted by many to register dismay for anything and everything. And I'll let you in on a not-too-secret secret: Most doctors get a symbolic backache (or headache) whenever someone comes in with a complaint of low back pain. It's a tough problem.

The list of conditions which can cause low back pain is almost endless. Conditions in the abdomen or pelvis, for example, commonly cause back pain. But the most common causes of true back disease are muscle strain, arthritis, congenital deformities of the spine, and disk disease. I will, therefore, confine my discussion to these major problems.

Muscle Strain

Our backs are loaded with muscles large and small. Given the manner in which we have defied our ancestry (by audaciously assuming the upright position) and the ways in which we daily abuse our backs, it is a wonder that we don't have more "back strain." Understand that the strain involved is that of muscles—not of the bony structure itself. And, like all muscle strain, treatment consists of heat, rest, and pain medicine when necessary; muscle-relaxant drugs are widely used, but their effectiveness (apart from time and rest) is not clearly established.

Prevention is the key—which means learning to lift by bending our knees rather than bending at the waist. And some specialists are now saying that the "slump" position, so long the object of mother's ire, is not so bad for the back; it may in fact be "restful" for the back. (Is nothing sacred anymore?) Finally, it should be mentioned that firm abdominal muscles (remember sit-ups?) seem to be an excellent guard against back trouble.

Arthritis

It is critical that you understand two things: (1) Most arthritis of the back is of the "natural" or "aging" variety, and (2) arthritis seen on X rays is not always significant.

There are two major forms of arthritis, osteoarthritis and rheumatoid arthritis. Rheumatoid disease is a systemic disease, that is, it affects several joints and possibly other organs and usually involves other symptoms such as fever, fatigue, etc. Osteoarthritis, on the other hand, is more of a local, mechanical-wear-and-tear process that is very common as we grow older. It is this kind of arthritis which most commonly affects the backbones. Unfortunately there is little that can be done about this kind of arthritis except surgical intervention when the process is so severe as to merit such drastic treatment; for example, arthritic changes of the spine—particularly in the neck—may impinge on the spinal cord enough to warrant surgery.

Fortunately, most arthritic change of the spine does not pose such serious problems. Indeed, some X rays of the spine may look "terrible" without the patient having any symptoms—and vice versa. I mention this because too often a person will be told that his spine shows "arthritic changes" (on X rays taken for other reasons) and that individual will then worry about his back falling apart. If it doesn't hurt, don't worry about it.

Congenital Deformities

Many people (younger people in particular) go to see the doctor with a backache and come out with a diagnosis consisting of an unpronounceable word—spondylolysis or spondylolisthesis. These words (and others) refer to defects in the bony structure of the spinal column which have been present since birth. Such defects usually are not discovered until later life—usually late teens or early adulthood—when the abnormal posture or motion resulting from such deformities may manifest with back pain.

It is very difficult to correlate such deformities as seen on X rays with actual symptoms. If symptoms are very severe then surgery may have to be considered. But most of the pain that caused X rays to be taken will get better with appropriate rest, after which specific exercises (Williams's exercises) may be helpful.

Disk Disease

We now come to the most common and controversial of the causes of severe low back and leg pain. A little anatomy lesson is required.

The *spinal column* is composed of a series of individual bones (vertebrae) held together by ligaments and separated by disk-shaped cushions logically called intervertebral disks. These disks separate and cushion the bulky parts of the vertebrae. Arch-shaped bones extend from the bulky parts of the vertebrae to form a posterior canal down which the *spinal cord* extends from the brain. From this cord, nerves extend out between the vertebrae to supply the parts of the body including the arms and legs. If the disk material pushes out from between the vertebrae into the spinal cord or the nerves extending from it, symptoms will be produced—pain, weakness, numbness, etc.—in the areas served by that part of the cord or the nerves extending from it at that level. This is what happens in disk disease. This pushing of the disk against the cord and/or nerves can be caused by a sudden rupture or by gradual weakening of the structure of the disk.

A careful examination is required to determine just what level of the spinal cord is involved; the distribution of the symptoms will usually signal the given disk involved. Two other diagnostic aids—in addition to back X rays—are often used. First is the *Myelogram,* which involves injecting dye (sometimes air) into the space surrounding the spinal cord, thus outlining areas where the disk is pushing on the cord or nerves. This procedure involves only minor risk when done by trained physicians, and it adds greatly to diagnostic information. I am going to go out on a limb and suggest that (almost) never should surgery for disk disease be done without a myelogram first being done to demonstrate that disk disease is indeed responsible for given symptoms. A myelogram is done with local anesthesia and is usually almost painless. *Discograms* involve injection of dye directly into the disk, which represents a more direct way of demonstrating where the disk is. However, this procedure is more difficult and therefore involves greater risk; it is not routinely done for disk problems.

Neither of these procedures, it should be emphasized, is

a substitute for careful history and physical examination, but the myelogram is very important to final diagnosis.

We now come to the question of surgery for disk disease. There is no question that unnecessary back surgery is done too commonly to ignore the problem. There are two problems with such surgery: (1) Like any unnecessary surgery, unnecessary risk and expense are involved, and (2) such surgery may not solve the problem and often makes it worse. The only way to avoid unnecessary surgery is to seek competent evaluation and advice *and ask questions:* Will the surgery help? (No one can give a guarantee but the asking of the question will put the recommending physician on proper alert.) Will the surgery be better than waiting and treating with rest, traction, etc.? Will you show me the anatomical problem on the myelogram (which should be done if surgery is being recommended)? There is no easy guideline—except to ask these and similar questions.

Disk surgery is performed by both orthopedic surgeons and neurosurgeons in this country. A debate between the two as to which can best do such surgery is usually lively; the orthopedist argues that he best knows how to take care of the back, and the neurosurgeon argues that he best understands the anatomy of the spinal cord and nerves. Actually, who does what in a given area is usually a matter of local medical politics which often boils down to who got "control" in a given hospital first. Either can do the surgery if properly trained.

Within the past few years, considerable attention has been given to "disk injections" for treatment of disk disease. This is the only major development in the treatment of disk disease in the past forty years. As of this writing, disk injection treatment (which involves injection of chymopapain directly into the disk to "shrink and dissolve" it) has not been approved for general use by the FDA. It has, however, received considerable experimental use, with over 12,000 injections having been done in this country. The major problem to date has been the development of both immediate and delayed (up to two weeks) sensitivity reactions. For this reason—and because of the technical skill required—the procedure is being done in the operating room under general anesthesia. The results to date have indicated about ninety percent effectiveness in properly selected cases; the procedure seems to be most effective in the relief of leg pain secondary to compression of the nerves by the disk. There has been considerable controversy surrounding the safety of the material injected; some of this controversy has had political overtones and has included opposition by neurosurgeons, since orthopedists have taken the lead in developing the procedure. The American Academy of Orthopedic Surgeons is in the midst of a training program for 2400 of its members so that, when and if the FDA approves the procedure, doctors properly trained will be available. The procedure is not applicable to all disk problems, but in suitable cases it presents a significant alternative to surgery.

Low Back Pain Doctors
Though I have commented on the involvement of orthopedists and neurosurgeons in the treatment of disk disease, I have not talked about what kind of doctor is best for initial diagnosis and treatment of low back pain. Either an orthopedist or neurosurgeon will have expertise applicable for such problems. However, for routine back strain problems, any primary care physician—or emergency room physician—should be qualified to sort out strain from more serious problems. This "sorting out"

should involve careful examination (touching, raising legs, checking reflexes, etc.). Back X rays need not be done if the pain is obviously a muscle strain. If the cause of the pain is not clear or if it has become a recurrent problem and no X rays have been done previously, then X rays are in order; such X rays should be avoided if at all possible in a woman who might be pregnant, since they do involve a more than average dose of radiation.

Baldness (*Alopecia*)

As in many areas of skin problems, the official terminology is extensive and confusing. But for practical nonprofessional purposes, loss of hair may be divided into two major categories; hair loss that is "natural" (due to heredity, without known cause) and hair loss which is secondary to some disease or irritant and therefore potentially reversible. Unfortunately, most hair loss cannot be reversed. Which leaves three options:

1. *Accept it:* Easy to say for those of us who have full heads (of hair). There are compensations. Many women find bald men attractive, and the saving of time and money on hair care is significant.

2. *Try snake oil:* It won't work—but there is no scientific evidence that anything else will either. Now I'm not going to go on record and say that hair growth has not coincided with some one of the thousands of home remedies that have been tried over the years, and if you want to waste time and money go ahead—as long as you can make sure that whatever is tried won't ruin what hair you have left, or the scalp now open to view.

3. *Surgery—hair transplant:* This is a legitimate—and expensive—way to cover bald areas. The surgery involves

taking hair from areas where it won't be missed and transplanting such hair (either in strips or more commonly in small, round punches) to areas where it *is* missed. No question that this works for the short run. But the long-term questions have not yet been answered: Will the transplant hair survive indefinitely? If it doesn't, what will that area look like—a scarred battlefield? Whether this kind of treatment is for you depends more on social and financial than medical considerations. It is safe and effective (though we don't know the long-term results) when performed by a competent physician—usually a plastic surgeon or a dermatologist. Unfortunately, some incompetent physicians have started to do hair transplants without adequate training and experience (the money is good and quick) so check the track record and training of the doctor who is going to scalp you.

4. If all else fails, wigs natural-looking enough to fool your barber are available everywhere.

Bed-Wetting (*Enuresis*)

The possible causes of unintentional urination are many and include the full range from general physical disease (diabetes) to specific urinary tract problems (bladder neck abnormalities) to functional (emotional) disturbances. True enuresis is unintentional urination for which no gross urinary tract problem can be found.

Most children are toilet trained by the age of three; boys take longer. By age five, only fifteen percent of boys and ten percent of girls are wetters; by age nine, the percentage has dropped to five. Toilet training should never be forced; it occurs naturally in the vast majority of children

The most important statement I can make about wetting is that it should always be approached as a sign of possible organic disease and should never be approached as a sure sign of psychological trouble. The latter may turn out to be the case, but it should be a conclusion reached only after careful exclusion of other causes. In the absence of obvious anatomical problems (difficulty starting or maintaining urination, etc.) or a diurnal pattern of wetting (wetting during the daytime as well as at night), most pediatricians feel that a urinalysis and culture to check for infection is all the testing that should be done. Many experts now feel that the most common cause of enuresis is "deep sleeping" in which the child is unresponsive to stimuli from a full bladder; this type of enuresis will often be responsive to Tofranil (a mood-elevating drug for adults) and/or conditioned reflex training (using alarm devices). But the passage of time usually takes care of the problem.

Most pediatricians are "tuned in" to this problem—but if yours is not, seek the advice of a urologist. (If you cannot easily find one, call the nearest teaching hospital and ask about a pediatric urologist in your area.) Surgery is seldom necessary; beware of a urologist who quickly, and without careful examination and explanation, recommends surgery.

Contraception (*Birth Control*)

The freedom to prevent conception is one of the prominent achievements of modern science. The sale and demonstration of birth control devices and/or medications is legal in all fifty states. All religious faiths endorse family planning, though the Roman Catholic church still officially requires that this be accomplished by abstinence. Despite such significant scientific and social advances, however, the perfect form of contraception does not exist. All present forms have disadvantages, and a choice of contraception requires thoughtful consideration of all possibilities by both physicians and users. The following represents a survey of currently available contraceptive methods with a highlighting of relative effectiveness and important dangers. The listing is done in order of effectiveness.

Sterilization Procedure

Vasectomy in the male and tubal ligation in the female are surgical procedures which mechanically interrupt the pathways for sperm and eggs, thereby preventing union and conception. As such, they are almost always permanent (irreversible) forms of contraception, though such procedures may occasionally be successfully reversed with a second operation. However, no one should have such a procedure done with the expectation that it can be reversed; a decision to have a sterilization procedure must include the overwhelming likelihood of permanency. There are experimental efforts to introduce "two-way valves" into sterilization procedures making later pregnancy possible, but these procedures are not yet available to the general public.

The details of sterilization are too complex—both medically and psychologically—to discuss in this book: It is imperative that thorough discussion between all parties involved be done *before* the surgery—after is too late. I would, however, mention two minor controversies related to vasectomies.

First, several years ago an academic urologist (medical

school professor) suggested that vasectomies might cause later health problems of an "autoimmune" nature—i.e., problems related to the body's reaction to its own tissues. While it must be honestly said that we do not fully know the long-term consequences of vasectomy, these suggestions have not been substantiated or supported by other urologists, and vasectomies are considered to be as safe as any minor surgical procedure. There can indeed be post-operative problems (bleeding, infection, etc.), but these are rare and only very rarely serious. One way to minimize such operative risks is to have the procedure done by a surgeon (both general surgeons and urologists do them) who has experience with the anatomy of the area; vasectomies should not be done by a physician who does them only rarely.

Second, some men have put sperm on ice before having a vasectomy. To be more specific, specimens of semen— the fluid ejaculated during sexual intercourse—can be stored indefinitely at very low temperatures; such "sperm on ice" can later be used for artificial insemination in order to achieve conception. I am not recommending that this be done (for one thing, it is expensive), but as yet such a procedure does not seem to endanger resultant offspring and it seems in other ways to be medically feasible.

One final word. Don't count on sterilization procedures for contraception until the doctor performing the surgery verifies the effectiveness with appropriate tests. Usually a period of several weeks is required before the surgical results cause effective contraception.

Birth Control Pills (*Hormonal Suppression of Ovulation*)
"The pill" has revolutionized birth control both medically and psychologically. Since clinical trials were first started

in 1954, the use of the pill has been the subject of many controversies, some of which continue even today. Nevertheless, it remains a widely used form of contraception and, when used appropriately, represents the most effective form of pregnancy prevention (except sterilization).

A survey of the varieties and combinations of pills available is beyond the scope of this book. Two points concerning pill choices should, however, be made.

The first point to note is that one of the reasons that the pill should be prescribed only after thoughtful examination is that birth control pills do differ in terms of side-effects; often these can be predicted beforehand and "the right pill for the right woman" can be selected if a careful medical history is taken. Then, too, a woman who experiences troubling side-effects from a given pill should not conclude that the pill is not for her. If there are good reasons for her to take the pill as a form of contraception, she should discuss the problems with her doctor. More often than not, another pill can be selected which will not present side-effects. But this requires communication between the woman involved and a doctor who is thoroughly familiar with the various pills; usually this means a gynecologist versus a generalist or internist.

We are now ready to discuss in more detail some of the more significant side effects and/or concerns regarding the pill. Here goes:

Does the pill cause cancer? The only honest answer is that there is no evidence *to date* that the pill causes cancer. Even more specifically, there is no evidence that the pill causes cancer of the breast, cancer of the uterus (endometrium), or cancer of the cervix. Indeed, there *may* be a protective effect of the pill against the development of endometrial cancer, since the pill promotes a thorough shedding of the endometrium. This is not to say that in the future some link between the pill and cancer might not be discovered; it is simply to say that *to date* there is no such evidence.

Women who have had certain breast tumors (which are estrogen dependent) or fibroids of the uterus probably should not take the pill since the pill may promote further growth of such abnormal tissues (versus *causing* such abnormalities). Some authorities use a low-estrogen-potent progestin pill in patients with small fibroids, but careful followup is mandatory.

There is considerable confusion about "vaginal cancers in young girls caused by hormones." The facts, in brief, are these: DES (diethylstilbestrol), a synthetic hormone used during the 1950s in an attempt to prevent miscarriage, has been clearly linked to the development of rare vaginal cancers in the daughters of women who were so treated. Note carefully that these hormones were given in large amounts to women *who were pregnant*—which is entirely different than use of the pill, which is designed to *prevent pregnancy*. For several reasons, physicians are increasingly reluctant to use any medications—including hormones—during the early stages of pregnancy. And this is one reason why careful examination (in this case to make sure the woman is not pregnant) should be part of any pill prescribing; it should not be simply "handed out."

Does the pill cause blood clots? The answer is that there is an increased risk of blood clot formation while taking the pill but that such a risk is minimal. There is no question now that women taking the pill have an increased risk of clot formation and therefore an increased risk of some of the complications of clots such as strokes. However, this risk is very small; for example, one reliable study indicates that risk of death from clots in pill users is about 1.5 to 4 per 100,000 as against 0.4 per 100,000 in nonusers. This must all be put in perspective by pointing out that the risk of death from pregnancy (which is what the pill is designed to "prevent") is about 21 per 100,000.

Does the pill cause birth defects? A recent issue of the prestigious *New England Journal of Medicine* again raised this question by reporting a study suggesting a possible association between the pill and limb abnormalities in off-spring. An accompanying editorial pointed out that we do not have good answers to this important question and that it is hoped that large studies now underway will pro-vide answers. In the meantime, pill users should be as-sured that, if such an associated risk does exist, it is a small one. Certainly women should make sure they are not pregnant before taking the pill, and it might be wise to suggest that pregnancy be delayed with other forms of contraception for several months after stopping the pill. Also, hormonal pregnancy tests should not be used.

Does the pill decrease subsequent fertility? (In other words, can you get pregnant after taking the pill?) The answer is, "Yes, you can get pregnant after the pill is stopped." About three-fourths of all pill users will get pregnant within two months after stopping the pill if no other means of contraception is substituted.

Certain women—as is obvious from the above discussion —should not take the pill. Avoid the pill if you have:

1. A history of breast cancer or other female cancers

2. A history of stroke or other evidence of clot-type disease

3. A history of other vascular disease—migraine head-aches, "poor circulation," etc.

4. A history of liver disease (the pill affects liver function) or gallstones

5. Severe diabetes (the pill affects sugar metabolism)

6. Large fibroids of the uterus (the pill may cause them to enlarge)

A quick word about two other kinds of pills—the "mini-pill" and the "morning after" pill. The "mini-pill" is a pill composed of low-dose progestins, one of the two major kinds of hormones used in most birth control pills. Since the other major kind of hormone, estrogen, is thought to be responsible for most of the serious side-effects associated with the pill, this kind of pill is obviously an attempt to reduce such possibilities. This type of pill is thought to act by making the cervix (the opening to the womb) hostile to sperm. Its two major problems are a slightly increased chance of pregnancy (versus other more traditional pills) and an increased incidence of "break-through" bleeding and menstrual irregularities. But it is an excellent alternative for those women who cannot tolerate the estrogen content of other pills.

The "morning after" pill is simply an estrogen taken for several days after intercourse; the hormone acts in this instance to prevent implantation of a possibly fertilized egg in the womb. The estrogen ordinarily used, DES, is the same one discussed above as related to vaginal cancer in female offspring when they reach the age of puberty. Other estrogens have recently been used instead of DES.

Finally, a word about injectable hormone contraception. Depo-Provera, an injectable form of progesterone, was temporarily approved by the FDA for use as an intramuscular injection every three months; as of this writing, such approval has been withdrawn. One of the problems with this approach has been delayed ovulation and consequent infertility; this usually can be corrected with the use of Clomid, a commonly used fertility drug.

In summary, then, the pill represents an excellent form of pregnancy prevention. The extremists on both sides have done a disservice to women who wish to use this form of contraception. Those who paint unwarranted "scare scenarios" produce fear which makes intelligent consideration impossible. Those who ignore the real dangers for certain women do the same.

IUD'S (*Intrauterine Devices*)

These are plastic or metal devices of many shapes and forms which are inserted by means of a sterile tubelike device into the womb; such insertion is easiest just after the menstrual flow when the cervix is somewhat dilated. The actual method by which pregnancy is prevented is not known, though most feel that the lining of the uterus is affected in a manner which prevents implantation of a possibly fertilized egg.

IUD's are slightly less effective than the pill but, along with the pill, they are clearly superior to other forms of contraception. Their major drawback is a fairly large number of side-effects (about twenty percent) which require the removal of the IUD within the first two to three months of insertion; most common are abdominal cramps and/or excessive bleeding. Another major problem is spontaneous expulsion (i.e., they fall out); if this goes undetected the woman is at obvious risk of pregnancy.

Recently the Dalkon Shield IUD received considerable publicity when the FDA ordered it off the market after reports of serious infection *during pregnancy* with the IUD still in place. It should be emphasized that the Dalkon was identified in this problem *only* when pregnancy occurred. Certainly Dalkon IUD's should be removed as soon as pregnancy is diagnosed. Some gynecologists are recommending their removal even before that possibility (and the insertion of another IUD).

It should also be stated that most gynecologists recommend the removal of any IUD if pregnancy occurs. Many pregnancies have been completely successful with an IUD left in, but a foreign body in the womb during pregnancy may be troublesome. Usually the removal will not cause an "abortion," since implantation generally occurs above the IUD.

For most women, then, an IUD is a good form of contraception—minimal in continuing cost and requiring no daily effort or concern.

Other Forms of Contraception

Three other forms of contraception can be grouped together as being considerably less effective than the pill or an IUD, but certainly much better than the rhythm method. A major problem with all of the following is that they require mechanical activity before intercourse, which therefore interferes with lovemaking.

Diaphragms and jellies: This method, when careful fitting and strict use occur, is quite effective; the diaphragm without a spermatocidal vaginal jelly or cream is less effective. This method does present a reasonable alternative for the woman who cannot use either the pill or IUD. Some women find the only way to use this method safely is to insert the diaphragm each night as a matter of habit whether or not sexual activity occurs.

Foams and jellies alone: Better than nothing but not as effective as the other methods.

Condoms and jellies: These coverings of the penis afford protection roughly equal to the diaphragms and jellies. They also afford some protection against venereal disease.

The condom remains the most common form of contraception worldwide. Its disadvantages are cost, inconvenience, and mechanical problems including tearing or leaking.

Rhythm Method

The old joke in medical school is that people who use the rhythm method are called parents. There is great truth in this, but the dismissal of this method so easily does disservice to those who for religious or other reasons must use this form of family control. While this approach to contraception will never be good, the chances can be improved by serious attempts to avoid the fertile period. In a woman with irregular cycles, this is almost impossible. But with regular cycles, several calculations are available to attempt to pinpoint the fertile period. Attention to basal body temperature may also be useful. Careful instruction by a knowledgeable contraception expert is essential in applying these methods. It should be pointed out that sperm escape from the penis during the excitation phase before actual ejaculation; thus, pregnancy can occur if the penis is in the vagina even though it is withdrawn before ejaculation.

Summary

Contraception is a complex medical and social arena requiring sound and sympathetic advice. It is important for a couple desirous of preventing pregnancy to seek sound counsel. Not every physician is capable of such. Often a family planning clinic (such as Planned Parenthood) offers the best source of complete advice without prejudice. No woman should use any form of contraception without first undergoing a thorough history and physical examination to make sure that a given method is appropriate for her. Where this is absolutely impossible the use of the condom by the male represents the best method of contraception without medical advice.

The ideal form of contraception—completely safe *and* effective—is not "just around the corner." Very likely such contraception will be local in action rather than involve systemic (affecting the whole body) medication. Considerable research is being done in areas such as "instant abortion" (inducing menstruation), male pills, immune mechanisms, etc. But, again, none of these methods is expected to revolutionize contraception in the next few years.

Dental Care

Care of teeth has become a major health theme in our generally affluent society. I say this because traditionally tooth care comes near the bottom of health concerns when cost is a consideration. Unfortunately, too many people in our society cannot afford good dental or medical care; dentistry is often a greater *direct* financial burden, since office dentistry (which constitutes the bulk of dental care) is usually not covered by traditional health insurance policies. Indeed, this lack of dental care coverage is one health problem that needs a quick remedy; in the meantime, clinics associated with dental schools, government care centers, etc., will have to fill the gap.

Since I am not a dentist, I cannot comment on dental problems in any authoritative way. I will, however, list three of the most important and basic items of teeth care that we should all be aware of.

First of all, there is *fluoride,* which is the single most important preventive available for early tooth care. And fluoride in the water supply is the best way of accomplishing fluoride protection. Children experience a sixty to seventy percent reduction in new cavities when their water is fluoridated. Yet less than fifty percent of the nation's water supplies are fluoridated, resulting in an estimated $1,400,000,000 (yes, $1.4 *billion*) worth of unnecessary dental work. There is absolutely no good evidence to suggest that water fluoridation in the amounts suggested by dental authorities (approximately one part per million) is dangerous.

In the absence of water fluoridation, other methods may be used. The next best methods are fluoridated vitamins and direct application of fluoride on the teeth by a dentist. (You should consult your dentist about these additional sources of fluoride even if your water is fluoridated.) Toothpastes with fluoride are certainly better than pastes without it but are no substitute for the methods just described.

Preserving "baby teeth" is another area whose importance we are now aware of. Baby teeth should be kept healthy until they fall out naturally; such preservation helps assure proper spacing and healthy development for the permanent teeth. Most dentists advise starting dental care no later than three years; some advocate regular checks as soon as teeth come in. Certainly the same concerns we should have for adult teeth—brushing, cavity repair, immediate attention to broken teeth, etc.—apply to baby teeth.

Adult tooth care, too, is an important item. Brushing and flossing are essential for tooth care at any age, but they become even more important in adults in order to prevent the most common cause of tooth loss in adults—

gum (periodontal) disease. Generally, cavities become less of a problem as we grow older, but gum disease increases. The effect of gum disease is to weaken the supporting soft tissue and bones in which teeth are "set." This in turn leads to tooth loss. And the best prevention against gum disease is brushing (carefully and systematically) and flossing to get at those areas that cannot be brushed; a dentist who does not instruct patients in these techniques is not practicing modern dentistry. Disclosing tablets (which can be purchased without prescription in any drugstore) are useful in identifying areas of plaque (the junk that needs to be brushed away). Water picks are no substitute for brushing and flossing but may be a useful addition to total tooth care. Signs of early gum disease include bleeding after brushing and red, puffy gum tissue; if your dentist thinks it advisable, he will suggest these be investigated by a periodontist for possible repair and restoration.

If ever prevention was a key word, it is so in tooth care —from the first tooth to gum care in adult life. And given the cost of dental care—which is usually out of pocket rather than covered by insurance—prevention makes very good economic sense.

Diabetes

This common disease (which affects three to four percent of our population) is too complex for a thorough discussion in this book. There are, however, certain areas of controversy—particularly treatment—which merit attention. Also worthy of stress is information concerning diagnosis and complications. These three sections are treated separately below.

Before turning to these sections, the following brief summary of the disease we call diabetes is in order.

1. Diabetes is typically described as a "disorder of glucose metabolism"—which is a fancy way of saying that sugar in the blood is not controlled and used in a normal way, usually due to deficiencies in insulin production. The more we study diabetes, the more we realize how much we don't know. The definition I have just given is very much oversimplified, but for our purposes it will do.

2. There is good evidence to suggest that there are two types of diabetes—a true deficiency of insulin (usually associated with diabetes in children) and the kind that is usually found in adults where lack of insulin is usually not the major problem. Treatment of these two forms obviously should be and is different.

3. The danger of diabetes is not primarily in the elevated levels of blood sugar (though, if extreme, such elevations can indeed be life-threatening), but in the long-term complications associated with diabetes. I deliberately say "associated with" rather than "caused by" to pinpoint a controversy that I will discuss more fully below.

Now we're ready to proceed to some specific areas of discussion.

Diagnosis

Most people are familiar with "urine screening" as a way of detecting diabetes. Due to the relative ease of obtaining and testing urine, this still remains an excellent screening method. However, actual diagnosis of diabetes requires blood testing, since "false positives" are possible with urine testing and many persons with mild diabetes will be missed.

A single blood test is not sufficient to diagnose diabetes. (The exception to this is a markedly elevated blood sugar level in a single test taken after fasting—i.e., first thing in the morning before eating.) Usually required is a glucose toler- ance test (GTT), which requires drinking of a heavy sugar liquid (or eating a meal rich in carbohydrates), followed by urine and blood samples taken at half-hourly and hourly intervals for up to five hours after drinking the liquid. The GTT will demonstrate various stages and patterns of diabetes, all of which are treated differently. It should also be mentioned that there are other tests which may be necessary to determine more fully the "sugar metabolism" status of the patient and to rule out diseases which mimic diabetes.

So much for the tests. The question remains: Who should have what tests—and when? Certain persons are at higher risk for the development of diabetes and should have blood tests taken more routinely than the general population. These high-risk persons include:

1. Persons with a strong history of diabetes. By "strong" I mean close relatives—parents, grandparents, and siblings. If both parents have diabetes, the chances of their children getting it are high.

2. Obese adults.

3. Women who give birth to very large babies or who have had mild diabetes during a pregnancy. Other women can rely on intermittent urine testing in the absence of symptoms.

Finally I come to symptoms. I have deliberately left this until last because most cases of adult diabetes do not present clear symptoms. Diabetes in children is usually more severe and exhibits more obvious warning symptoms

—excessive thirst and urination, increased appetite coupled with weight loss, night wetting, etc. Unfortunately, the diagnosis in children is still too often made only when severe illness (including coma) develop.

All of this is to say that the best method of diagnosis is a high index of suspicion coupled with accurate blood tests. Most physicians and lay people are alert to diabetes, but occasionally a severe case develops (especially in kids) before the diagnosis is made.

Treatment

First, some generalizations are in order. Most diabetes which starts in early childhood requires life-long insulin treatment; there are very few exceptions. On the other hand, many who develop diabetes in later years can be treated effectively with diet and weight modifications. Finally, those who develop diabetes in late childhood or early adulthood tend to fall in between regarding the severity of their diabetes.

Those who develop diabetes early in childhood are described as "juvenile diabetics." This phrase is more than a chronological label. It implies diabetes which is usually more severe, more "labile" (has marked swings in blood sugar and therefore in insulin requirements), and which, quite frankly, demands much more careful attention if a normal life is to be possible. Such diabetics must have medical attention involving exquisite attention to both physical and psychological needs.

Having offered these generalizations, I would like to examine certain treatment problems under the following categories:

Insulin: The subject of insulin treatment is very complex and, again, a full discussion is way beyond the scope of this book. Any person requiring insulin *must* be carefully instructed as to its use and dangers. Fortunately, most medical professionals who deal with diabetics are "tuned in" to the need for careful and continual instruction. But, if you are a diabetic and find your sources of care unresponsive, look elsewhere. Such instruction is too vital a part of treatment to be minimized.

Insulin measurement has been greatly simplified by the development of U100 syringes and concentrations. It should be emphasized that this insulin is the same as the U40 or U80 forms; it is just a different concentration making the measurement of appropriate doses less prone to error.

Patients who have been on insulin for years without difficulty may suddenly develop a change in their insulin requirements. There are many possible reasons for this (including so-called "insulin resistance"), but usually such a change implies a change in the health status of the individual which merits immediate investigation.

Oral drugs: We now come to a much more controversial subject. In 1970 a group of distinguished physicians (called the UGDP—the University Group Diabetes Program) published results suggesting that not only were oral drugs for diabetes ineffective in certain patients but also that they were dangerous to the cardiovascular system (heart and vessels). Specifically, this group suggested that one typical oral drug (Tolbutamide) is no more effective than diet in treatment and that, if more than diet is required, insulin should be used. They also suggested that a fixed-dose treatment with this drug was associated with a higher death rate from cardiovascular causes than diet alone or diet and insulin combined. That report provoked a response of marked disagreement from a group of equally distinguished physicians who argued with the method and results of the study and who further argued that oral drugs have a legitimate role in the treatment of certain diabetics. The Federal Food and Drug Administration responded to this confusing argument between experts by *recommending* (not demanding) that Tolbutamide and other sulfonylurea-type drugs should be limited to patients with symptomatic adult diabetes uncontrollable with careful diet and weight loss and unsuitable for insulin treatment. The controversy was recently refueled by the release of an NIH (National Institutes of Health) commissioned review of the original study; the review (reported in the February 10, 1975, issue of the *Journal of the AMA*) supported the original conclusions but those who initially disagreed with the findings still disagree. My own personal view—and I clearly identify it as such—is that the burden of proof has shifted to those who would prescribe oral pills for diabetes. At the very least, any patient taking such pills should discuss the matter thoroughly with his physician.

Diet: We are now in a better position to say that diet has been both overstressed and understressed. For the diabetic on insulin, severe diet restrictions are not as essential as has been suggested in the past. On the other hand, for the mild adult diabetic, careful attention to sugar intake may be all that is necessary to keep the blood sugar within acceptable range. Again, it is obvious that individualization is necessary.

Other factors: Attention to other details of treatment may make the difference between a normal and enjoyable life and one filled with upsets. Such details are subject to individual differences, but a brief listing will remind any diabetic of the possibilities:

- *Exercise:* Since exercise burns up sugar, insulin requirements may change when exercise levels change significantly. It is not unusual for a diabetic on large amounts of insulin to become hypoglycemic after strenuous exercise and most learn to fortify themselves beforehand. When insulin regulation is determined in a hospital setting, it is important to anticipate out-of-hospital activity levels.

• *Infections:* Infections are still the most common precipitating cause of diabetic coma (except omission of insulin) since infections generally increase insulin requirements. Any infection in the diabetic is potentially life-threatening and must be treated early and vigorously. Foot care, for example, is stressed to prevent minor foot problems from developing into major disasters.

• *Weight control:* As stressed above, weight control may be sufficient treatment in the mild, adult-type diabetes not requiring insulin. But even for the diabetic requiring insulin, weight control usually makes treatment much easier.

Complications

The acute complications of diabetes result from excessive swings in blood sugar—either too high from lack of control or too low from too much control (too much insulin or, rarely, too much oral medication). Either state in excess leads to a state of mood changes progressing to unconsciousness, which may be life-threatening if not treated vigorously.

More difficult to discuss are the long-term complications of diabetes: premature atherosclerosis (so-called hardening of the arteries), neuropathies (malfunctioning of the nervous system causing pain in the extremities or diarrhea and bladder problems), eye diseases (including several problems that can lead to premature blindness), kidney disease, skin infections, etc. The difficulty in discussing such complications is this: There is considerable controversy about whether strict control prevents or minimizes the development of such complications.

Currently, some experts feel that control of blood sugar may "pay off" in reducing the complications from premature atherosclerosis as it affects heart (coronary) and peripheral circulation. Complications affecting the vessels of the eye (retinal disease) and kidney (Kimmelstiel-Wilson disease) seem to be more related to the degree of control, although some recent evidence suggests that these abnormalities of small blood vessels (microangiopathy) may precede the onset of diabetes and may be caused by a genetic defect.

I do not want to minimize the importance of control, but I must honestly suggest that rigid and strict control may not be as helpful as was once thought since it is impossible with current methods for insulin administration to mimic the constant control that occurs in nondiabetics whose insulin level is constantly changing according to minute-to-minute needs. There are many other reasons to achieve control, not the least of which is the possibility of a more enjoyable life free from the disturbances of a diabetic coma. But you should understand that the issue of complications is far from settled.

Ear Problems

The most common serious ear problems are hearing loss and ear infections; they are discussed below—along with the less serious but even more common problem of ear wax. All ear problems can be seen initially by a good primary care physician. However, most hearing problems and any persistent infection problem should be examined by an ear specialist—an ENT (ear, nose, throat) specialist, also called an otolaryngologist. Certainly any definitive statement about hearing loss and proposed treatment (including the statement that "nothing can be done") must be verified by a competent specialist.

Hearing Loss

There are two basic kinds of hearing loss—conductive and sensorineural. Since it is important that you have a "feel" for the difference between these, I am going to describe (*very* simply) the process of hearing as follows: (1). Sound waves enter the ear and "travel" through the ear canal (external ear) to the eardrum (tympanic membrane). (2). The sound waves cause the eardrum to vibrate, and the three small bones connected between the eardrum and the inner ear also begin to vibrate; this space between the eardrum and inner ear containing the three small bones is known as the middle ear. (A tube called the eustachian tube runs from the middle ear to the back of the throat; that tube is designed to keep the pressure in the middle ear at a proper level, and, if it gets closed off by infection or allergy, trouble results). (3). The sound waves from the bones of the middle ear are now transmitted to the fluid of the structures of the inner ear; the movement of this fluid sets up impulses in nerve endings of the inner ear which are transmitted by the auditory nerve to the brain, where the impulses are interpreted as sound. (The inner ear also contains structures that maintain our sense of balance; diseases of this area may produce symptoms we describe as dizziness, vertigo, spinning, loss of balance, etc.)

Interference with the passage of sound waves in steps 1 and 2 (in the outer and middle ears) produces so-called "conductive hearing loss"; diseases of the inner ear or auditory nerve leading to the brain cause so-called "sensorineural hearing loss." In general, conductive hearing losses are surgically correctable, while sensorineural losses are not. (The one exception is a small benign tumor of the auditory nerve—called acoustic neuroma—which may be surgically removed and thereby restore hearing, if correction is done early enough.) The vast number of sensorineural hearing losses can be helped by an appropriately selected and fitted hearing aid.

Obviously it is important to evaluate carefully the exact reason for hearing loss. And this requires the special skills of a specialist in ENT. (Such a specialist may use the skills of an Audiologist, a nonphysician trained in the special skills of testing for hearing problems.) Two warnings are appropriate at this point. First, when hearing loss is suspected, go to an expert for evaluation. This is one time when the higher cost of a specialist is worth it. Second, do *not* assume that nothing can be done for your "poor hearing." In particular, avoid the hearing aid salesman who pushes expensive aids without a careful evaluation by a specialist. It may be that an aid will be the answer to your problem, but it would be a tragedy to miss something more correctable.

At this point it is fitting to talk about prevention of hearing loss. Some forms of hearing loss cannot be prevented—particularly those of the "aging" variety. But four areas of prevention deserve mention:

1. *Infections:* It is important that ear infections be promptly and effectively treated, since hearing loss may result from lack of such treatment. (See next page.)

2. *Injury:* Be sure to have your hearing evaluated after any significant injury to the ear.

3. *Noise pollution:* There is now good evidence that prolonged exposure to significant noise (including amplified "music") may cause hearing loss; if you value your hearing, you should "check out" such situations to find out what the dangers are and what you might do to minimize damage.

Finally, a word to parents. Be suspicious of a child who does not respond to your voice or other sound stimuli; don't just assume the child is being ornery. Call such behavior to the attention of your pediatrician. It would be a shame to overlook a hearing problem when it might be easily corrected or to deprive a child with a severe sensorineural hearing loss of the specialized treatment necessary for language development.

Ear Infections

First, it is important to understand that infections can occur in any of the three parts of the ear—outer, middle, inner. Outer ear infections (otitis externa) refers to infections of the external ear canal—so-called "swimmer's ear," though such an infection can occur even if you haven't been swimming. Middle ear infections refer to infections of the space behind the ear drum where the small ear bones are located. And inner ear infections refer to infections of the structures deeper in the skull concerned with hearing and balance. The point here is that an "earache" may be due to infection in any of these areas and it is important to pinpoint the problem since treatment is quite different depending on location; usually a look in the ear with an otoscope is sufficient to make the distinction.

If the problem is the outer ear, drops alone are usually sufficient. If the problem is the middle ear, antibiotics and antihistamines (to open drainage from the middle ear to the throat via the eustachian tubes) are required. There are several different kinds of infection, but they must be adequately treated to prevent permanent hearing damage and the spread of the infection to more vital structures.

The natural course for a middle ear infection that is not treated is for pus and fluid to build up behind the eardrum to the point where the drum ruptures; in the days before antibiotics this would be the usual course of events. Spontaneous rupture of the ear drum in a patient properly treated with antibiotics is rare today. Myringotomy, which is an incision in the ear drum, is sometimes done if infection does not properly respond to antibiotics and/or with accompanying signs of mastoid (behind the ear) infection.

It is important that any child who has had an ear infection be checked after treatment is completed to make sure that the infection has cleared up; sometimes symptoms will disappear but fluid will remain. The insertion of tubes into the ear drum is usually done for those children who have persistent accumulation of fluid in the middle ear. Such children may suffer from hearing loss or from recurring infections not responsive to antibiotics. In other words, fluid in the ear without adequate drainage predisposes the child to middle ear infection. (Tubes may also be inserted in stubborn cases of persisting infection.)

Finally, if fluid accumulates in the middle ear of an adult, a careful examination of the openings in the back of the nose and throat must be done to rule out growths which may be blocking the usual drainage route.

Ear Wax (Cerumen)

Wax in the ears is like a ring around the collar. We all have it. Wax is produced by glands in the outer one third of the external ear canal. The natural course of events is for wax to be brought to the opening of the ear by the natural movement of skin out toward that opening. It is usually sufficient to wash out the opening of the ear canal. Water placed into the canal may soften the skin and cause infection.

Cotton-tipped swabs, bobby pins, matches, etc., only serve to disrupt this wonderful natural mechanism and in the process they often injure the delicate skin of the ear canal, which in turn may lead to infection.

Once wax has built up to the point of blockage, removal by a doctor or other trained person is usually necessary.

Emotional Illness

I am not a psychiatrist and this book makes no pretense at adequately dealing with the great amount of emotional upset so common in our society. However, I would like to deal with the following practical questions related to emotional (mental) illness.

How does one recognize mental illness? In many instances of disturbance, the signs are obvious—very strange behavior, hallucinations, thought processes that are "out of touch," etc. The asking of this question, however, points to the more common situation in which a person feels troubled, depressed, "strange"—but is not clearly "crazy." All of us have had moments when we wonder if we are "losing our minds." All of us worry about recognizing when a member of our family or circle of acquaintances "needs help."

The answer to this question is not easy since the range

of "normal" is so variable. Indeed, the definition of "normal behavior" can provoke intense discussion and disagreement among experts. But my concern here is not to satisfy the experts but to offer you a practical guide in answering this important question. And the guide that I find most useful is this one: A person needs help when his emotions interfere significantly with his ability to function. This answer stresses two words—*significant* and *function.* By "function" I mean those required activities of life—eating, sleeping, working, relating to other people. By significant I mean the degree of intensity (breakdown obviously describes an intense interruption in function) and the time element involved; even a relatively small change in functioning that persists should be cause for concern.

This kind of guideline avoids labels which are not very useful except to the expert. It does give us all a yardstick by which to measure ourselves and others. And it obviously allows for a wide range of "normalcy" in which differences of personality and style and choice are accepted as long as a person can function in terms of essentials. This guideline offers some objective signs of difficulty— the person who has persistent loss of appetite, who has new and persistent insomnia (particularly early awakening), who cannot do required work, who cannot handle schoolwork (presuming adequate I.Q.), who cannot relate to other people to the minimal degree required to get through a day, etc.

It should also be apparent that these manifestations of emotional illness may also be signs of a physical problem. One of the great tragedies of life and medical practice is that person who is "passed off" as being "disturbed" or "psychosomatic" when in fact serious underlying disease is the cause. (The other side of this coin is the person who cannot accept the possibility of a problem that is not physical; such persons are often "helped" by placebo treatments —vitamin shots, treatment for alleged hypoglycemia, etc.) Anyone demonstrating the "inability to function" deserves a good physical examination before being considered for treatment for emotional disturbance—which leads to the next logical question.

Who is best qualified to treat emotional disturbance? The obvious answer to that should be "a psychiatrist." You will recall that a psychiatrist has had standard medical training plus at least three years of residency in the diagnosis and treatment of emotional illness. Other mental health professionals may have had equally rigorous psychological training without the standard medical degree (clinical psychologists). Still others (psychiatric social workers, mental health nurses, etc.) have had lesser degrees of training.

It would appear that a psychiatrist could offer the best of both diagnostic worlds—medicine and psychology. However, many psychiatrists have separated themselves from traditional medical practice and rely on other physicians for physical examination and diagnosis. And, since the standards and skills of psychological therapy are much less standardized than those of traditional medicine, the selection of an appropriate therapist is very difficult. All of this is a long-winded way of saying that I can't really answer the question I have posed. Since the range of emotional illness is so great, the treatment resources are also varied.

I would suggest that you consider other resources than a yellow-page listing of psychiatrists. The mental health movement of our times has spawned many clinics based in churches, schools, neighborhood health centers, and so on. If these clinics are sponsored by reputable outfits, they often offer a greater range of service (at more reasonable prices) than the traditional private practitioner.

A good primary care physician is often an excellent guide to appropriate treatment resources. Many non-psychiatric physicians are skeptical of the personnel and treatment methods of psychiatry; unfortunately, they sometimes share this skepticism with patients who might benefit from such treatment. But this same skepticism has also caused many primary care physicians to search for reliable treatment facilities.

Another source of counsel should be the religious institutions of our society. Modern training for priests, rabbis, and ministers places heavy emphasis on counseling and mental health. For persons active in religious life, these resources should be explored.

What about the use of drugs and/or shock therapy? Tranquilizers are the most widely used drugs in our society—besides minor painkillers. There are two major classes of tranquilizers, minor and major.

The minor tranquilizers (Valium, Librium, Serax, etc.) are widely prescribed in our society. Every physician has anecdotal evidence to support their usefulness, but hard scientific evidence is harder to come by. They are relatively safe, though when taken in large amounts or in combination with alcohol (or other drugs) they can be lethal. My personal opinion is that their use should be restricted to times of temporary upset; chronic use usually indicates a problem worth exploring with a mental health professional.

Major tranquilizers (Thorazine, Mellaril, etc.) are much

more potent and are used for psychotic illness (e.g., schizo-phrenia) and severe agitation. Such drugs have restored many seriously ill people to relatively normal lives and have done much to decrease the need for institutionalization. Often persons requiring such drugs will need them for long periods of time and will regress if they stop taking them.

A quick word about barbiturate medications is in order. These are most commonly used for sleeping medication, but I would like to echo a recent editorial in the *New England Journal of Medicine* which suggests that these dangerous drugs should no longer be used for this purpose since we have more effective and less dangerous sleeping medication available.

One other drug should be mentioned: Lithium, which is used for manic depressive illness. This particular illness, marked by swings between depression and highs, responds to Lithium in a significant number of cases. Lithium is particularly effective in preventing the marked extremes of the illness. It is not effective in so-called monophasic depression—i.e., those depressions which do not alternate with highs.

Shock therapy is most effective in the depressive illnesses, particularly those related to "change of life" (so-called "involutional melancholia"). It has been abused in the past and applied to all kinds of emotional disturbances. A good primary care physician should be consulted before shock therapy is used.

What about "talking therapy"? Traditional psycho-therapy—talking to a mental health professional—has been under attack in recent years both for cost and questioned effectiveness. Most everyone, including mental health professionals, would agree that treatment methods are difficult to evaluate in the area of mental health. Problems in people who are articulate can often be helped by therapeutic conversation. If any long-term psychotherapy is proposed, you should question the proposal in terms of cost, expected results, time involved, etc.

In Summary
Objective information and advice is hard to come by in dealing with emotional disturbance. A good primary care physician is probably the best source of guidance to treatment options.

Eye Problems
I am lumping the most common eye problems together in one section to indicate that eyes are indeed a very special part of our anatomy, crucial to normal function and deserving of the special expertise of the ophthalmologist *whenever* there is any question as to danger to vision. This is one of those areas of medical concern where the main rule is: *Take no chances!*

Having said this, I am immediately aware of the frustration produced by the restricted availability and high fees of the typical ophthalmologist. Typically such frustration is produced when a person seeks a routine eye exam and is told that no appointment is available for many months. If the concern *is* routine and there is no symptom or change in vision to provoke concern, it is not unreasonable to wait for such an exam. If, however, there is cause for concern (and I'll define that shortly), you must become aggressive in insisting on proper care. Explain your concern by being specific as to what is bothering you. Put the doctor on the spot by indicating that you have fulfilled your responsibility by calling your concern to his attention. If this approach fails, go to an emergency facility which can evaluate you and which will have access to emergency eye care if needed.

Now: What is legitimate cause for concern? Certainly *any* of the following symptoms merits investigation: pain, blurred vision, discharge which is copious or pussy, persistent "spots before the eyes," double vision. Any of these may be a sign of serious disease requiring emergency treatment. Also, any injury to the eye (other than *very* minor incidents) should be evaluated quickly. And, finally, any foreign body in the eye which does not come out easily with normal tearing should be treated quickly; such foreign bodies are much easier to remove before they become "covered over" by new tissue growth in the eye.

As mentioned in the section on emergencies, I wish to stress one situation in which *your immediate treatment* (not the doctor's or hospital's) can make the difference between preservation of vision and loss of eyesight— namely, the splashing of any toxic material (such as acid or lye) into the eyes. The treatment for such an emergency is copious flushing of *water* into the eye by whatever means available—pouring (if assistance is available to pour and hold the eyelids open) or opening and closing the eyelids in a pan of water or the cupped hand. The water need not be sterile; the cleanest water available should be used. The emphasis is on speed, since the purpose of such flushing is to remove the irritant from the eye before permanent damage is done to the cornea (the clear area in the front of the eye through which light must pass for vision to occur). Only after a minimum of twenty minutes of such flushing should you make arrangements to go and have your eyes checked by your doctor or the nearest hospital emergency room.

We now come to the subject of pink eye. This is not only the most common eye symptom but also the most difficult for the average person to evaluate, since most pink eye is not serious, even though quite distressing. "Pink eye," of course, is a lay phrase referring to redness of the eye which may or may not involve other symptoms—pain, blurring of vision, etc. Certainly any redness of the eye which is accompanied by any of the serious symptoms I have just mentioned deserves a visit to the doctor. But, quite frankly, most "pink eye" turns out to be "viral conjunctivitis" (inflammation of the lining of the eye) which will get better with time; therefore, it is not unreasonable to wait several days with a pink eye that is mild and without any other symptoms.

A final word of warning: Never use eye medications without guidance from a doctor. It is incredible what people will put in their eyes without checking as to safety or appropriateness. Any eye medication that has been opened may become contaminated—especially stuff that has been lying around in a medicine cabinet for several years. Certain eye medications may cause permanent damage when used for the wrong conditions.

Glaucoma and cataracts are diseases of the eye which pose special problems and should be treated only by a fully trained eye specialist (ophthalmologist).

Cataracts

A cataract is a clouding of the lens of the eye which interferes with vision. The vast majority occur as a "natural" part of aging; indeed, most people over sixty have some degree of lens clouding. Two critical questions present to the person with cataracts: Should I have surgery? and What kind of surgery should I have?

The answer to the first question really boils down to one simple question: How much do cataracts interfere with the desired ability to function? If vision is compromised to the point where life becomes hampered (either in terms of safety or enjoyment), surgery should be strongly considered, since there is no other treatment for cataracts. If, however, the cataract does not interfere with functioning, there is no need to rush into surgery; there is no harm to the eye in waiting to see how the cataract progresses ("ripens").

Cataract surgery today is very safe, very effective, and involves little postoperative discomfort. However, persons undergoing such surgery should understand that their vision will not be restored to that of a teenager. It will be dramatically improved in most cases, but it will not be perfect. Strong lenses (either contact lenses or glasses) will be required after the operation to take the place of the damaged lenses removed in surgery. These qualifications should not frighten the person whose vision is impaired; cataract surgery is one of the great benefits of modern medicine.

Now comes the question of what kind of surgery. There are several different ways of destroying or removing the damaged lens. I will not presume to comment on which way is best, since the experts themselves cannot agree. When done correctly, they all seem to accomplish the job. You should ask your eye doctor to explain the various kinds of surgery available and to comment on his choice; if he sounds confident and reasonable, his choice should be accepted. After all, he wants a good result almost as much as you do.

Finally the question of cost. Cataract surgery is expensive—illogically so, in my estimation, when compared to other forms of surgery and medical treatment. Fortunately, most forms of insurance—including Medicare and Medicaid—will pay for such surgery. But when money is a real and honest problem lay it on the line with the eye surgeon you are dealing with. If he is any kind of decent human being, he will work out something satisfactory.

Glaucoma

Glaucoma is an eye disease difficult for the lay person to understand and therefore surrounded by misunderstanding. The most significant misunderstanding is the myth that glaucoma has clear warning signs which allow for treatment before damage is done. The fact is that, in the vast majority of cases, permanent loss of vision has occurred before any warning symptoms occur.

The basic problem posed by glaucoma is an increase in intraocular pressure (pressure within the eyeball) which damages the structures at the back of the eye responsible for vision. The only way to detect glaucoma in the early stages is to have your "eye pressure" checked whenever a good screening program is available and routinely as part of any physical exam past age forty. Pressure testing is done in several different ways, but all basically involve putting drops in the eye to render the surface of the eye insensitive to pain and then placing a small instrument on the eye to measure pressure. The procedure is safe and painless. It can be done by any person trained to do it; it does not have to be done by an ophthalmologist, though any abnormal results should be checked by one.

Having made the important point that glaucoma usually has no warning symptoms and can be detected only by pressure testing, I will now mention that a small number of cases (so-called "acute glaucoma") do present with severe symptoms: pain, blurring of vision, red eyes, cloudy cornea, etc. Such symptoms must be investigated immediately; there is no time to lose. Vision can be completely lost within days.

But symptoms are the exception. Most of the two million people with glaucoma in this country do not know they have it because they don't get their eye pressure checked. The stakes are too high to take a chance. When detected by pressure testing before loss of vision has occurred, glaucoma can be almost always successfully treated by medication; occasionally, surgery becomes necessary.

Fever

The basic question faced by someone with a fever is this: Does this fever mean that I am sick enough to seek medical attention? Since the fever provokes this kind of concern, it is important to make sure that the "body temperature" (which we call a fever when it is abnormally elevated) has been determined accurately. A temperature taken rectally is the most accurate—especially in children —and should be tried whenever there is a suspicion of the accuracy of the oral route.

The major point that should be made in the context of this book is that a given body temperature should not be used *alone* in making a decision as to whether or not to seek medical attention. This applies to both high and low fevers. For example, if a child acts sick (listless, vomiting, "just not right"), that child should be taken for examination even if the fever is low—as it often is with serious disease in the very young or very old. On the other hand, a person who feels and acts fine does not have to rush off to the doctor just because the oral temperature is 101° F.; if that temperature persists beyond twenty-four hours— even in the absence of symptoms—then a check is in order.

In other words, more important than any given temperature reading is the total medical situation; the "fever"— which is what most people worry most about—is only one clue as to the possible seriousness of the problem. And as mentioned above (it's worth repeating) body temperature is a less reliable sign of serious disease in the very young and very old. (In fact, other diagnostic signs—such as pain—are often less helpful in the young infant or the older person, which means that they should be checked more readily when things aren't "quite right.") If someone looks or acts or feels really sick—don't bother with a temperature. But, if someone has a fever less than 101° F. orally but feels fine otherwise, watchful waiting is in order —unless the person involved can't tell you how he feels or what might be bothering him.

The other basic question faced by someone with a fever is this: Can he take aspirin for a fever without checking with some medical source of information? Generally, if a person is otherwise healthy, is taking no other medications, and has had no previous difficulty with aspirin, it is legitimate to take the appropriate dose of aspirin for a simple fever—that is, with no other symptoms that merit checking. I say "generally" because we are much more aware of the dangers of aspirin than we used to be—particularly in persons with other illnesses (such as ulcers) or who are taking other medications (such as anticoagulants or "blood thinners"). Obviously a fever that cannot be easily controlled with aspirin or that continues to rise despite an appropriate amount of aspirin should be checked by a physician.

Genetic Counseling

My major purpose in writing this section is to explain what genetic counseling is—and is not. Genetic counseling is *not* an attempt to manipulate genes in order to produce superhuman offspring. "Genetic counseling" is just that— counseling which attempts to provide information to interested persons regarding the role of genes (heredity) in various health problems. Put specifically, it is an attempt to answer this common question: What are the chances of any child the parents might have being afflicted with a hereditary disorder? Variations on this question include concern for future children because of past birth defects, past family history, or certain concerns of age, race, etc.

The ability to answer these and related questions represents one of the great achievements of modern medicine. It is beyond the scope of this book to describe the complexities of modern genetics, but the following are among the most commonly asked questions concerning "hereditary disease."

What Is Meant by Hereditary or Genetic Disease?

In one sense, all disease might be described as hereditary —that is, any disease occurs in a specific human being with a specific genetic composition unique to that individual. But the phrase "hereditary disease" refers more specifically to diseases which are clearly caused by abnormal genes (such as mongolism—Down's syndrome) or abnormal metabolism (such as Tay-Sachs disease) that can be traced directly to parental genetic composition. Another practical way of defining genetic disease is as that disease which can be predicted by genetic counseling—see the next question.

Just What Is Involved in Genetic Counseling? Genetic counseling is usually done by pediatricians (or other physicians) with special training in the science of genetics. It is commonly available in teaching hospitals affiliated with medical schools, though it is becoming more common in community hospitals. The National Foundation (1275 Mamaroneck Ave., White Plains N.Y. 10605) and the National Genetics Foundation (250 W. 57th St., New York, N.Y. 10019) have lists of centers where adequately trained personnel can perform genetic counseling.

When a couple concerned about a current or future pregnancy requests answers to the kinds of questions described above, the genetic counselor will employ the following techniques in attempting to provide answers:

a. *Family history:* People seeking genetic counseling are often amazed at the detailed family information required. But often such careful history will be enough to provide the answers sought.

b. *Accurate diagnosis of past problems:* Sometimes the genetic counselor will request the opportunity to examine and study other family members in an attempt to be sure of accurate diagnosis of past problems.

c. *Screening studies:* Screening represents an attempt to detect genetic problems that are not otherwise obvious in a pair of prospective parents. The best known examples of such "hidden" problems are sickle-cell trait and Tay-Sachs disease, which happen to be more common in Black and Eastern European Jewish people, respectively. These kinds of diseases are described as "hidden" because, while the prospective parents appear to be perfectly healthy, they are "carriers" of abnormal genes which, if they combine in a certain way in a given offspring, will produce definite disease. The list of conditions which can be detected by screening blood and/or urine tests is growing each year.

Who Should Have Genetic Counseling?

This has become somewhat controversial. Obviously it would be difficult to provide thorough counseling to all prospective parents. Some have advocated screening as part of marriage license application, but that suggestion meets with criticism for obvious reasons. On an individual basis, however, the following groups of people should strongly consider some form of genetic counseling:

a. Persons with *specific disease problems* on either side of the family. Many diseases have no currently known hereditary component. But the only way to make sure is to ask a competent source of such information; usually a pediatrician is the best source. The two organizations mentioned earlier are good sources of information and further referral.

b. Persons of races or religions known to be a higher risk for certain diseases. Specifically, Black people (sickle-cell disease), Eastern European Jewish people (Tay-Sachs disease), and Mediterranean people (certain anemias) should seek advice and screening.

c. Persons with anxiety about future offspring may find counseling helpful.

How Can We Find Out if a Current Pregnancy Will "Turn Out O.K."?

We now come to the role of amniocentesis in genetic counseling. Amniocentesis is a procedure which involves inserting a long needle into the womb during pregnancy and through that needle obtaining fluid and cells from the fluid surrounding the developing fetus. (The lining of the womb in pregnancy is called the amnion and the fluid contained inside the lining is called the amniotic fluid— hence the name amniocentesis for the procedure.) Obviously the procedure involves some risks (infection, damage to the developing fetus, etc.), but the risks are minimal when done by well-trained individuals. This procedure can be used both to detect problems in the developing fetus and to follow a problem pregnancy (Rh disease, for example) to determine when intervention (transfusions, early delivery, etc.) might be needed. Aside from the problem pregnancy, the following groups of mothers should be considered for amniocentesis if they wish to consider the possibility of abortion to terminate a pregnancy which might result in an abnormal birth:

1. Partners with a history of previous abnormal births

2. Older pregnant women (the risk of Down's syndrome increases dramatically in pregnant women over age thirty-five)

3. Carriers of sex-linked diseases (hemophilia, for example)

4. Members of families with certain metabolic disorders (Tay-Sachs)

Obviously the answer to the question of who should undergo amniocentesis requires careful communication between a given woman and her obstetrician—and genetic counselors when needed. As in all of medicine, the questions come down to weighing relative risks and considering the full range of medical and social factors.

Again, this brief section can only give you a "feel" of what is involved in genetic counseling. Your best sources of detailed information are specific genetic counseling centers in your area.

German Measles (*Rubella*)

The importance of this disease lies in the damage that can be done to a developing fetus if a pregnant woman without immunity is exposed. The effects on a child or adult are almost always mild (unlike regular measles). Therefore, the focus of this discussion will be the potentially or actually pregnant woman.

Eighty percent of American women at age twenty are immune to rubella, which means they have been exposed to the disease during childhood and developed antibodies to the rubella virus. They may not have demonstrated the full-blown disease—general malaise, a fine rash of about three days' duration, swollen nodes in the back of the neck and behind the ear, etc.—but they had enough exposure to become immune. It is the other twenty percent that are at risk—or, to be more precise, whose possible children are at risk during pregnancy. A simple blood test can tell if immunity exists. Most obstetricians do such a blood test at the beginning of pregnancy; if immunity exists there is no worry about exposure during pregnancy, but if immunity does not exist any chance of exposure should be avoided.

For the woman entering child-bearing age who does not have immunity, the rubella vaccine should be given. (Mass immunization during childhood is now required in many states; the question that has been raised about such an approach is whether such immunity will last until adulthood and whether it would be better to allow natural exposure to occur, as it does in the majority of children.)

When the vaccine is given to such a woman, two things must be done. First, it must be established that the woman is not pregnant; and, second, careful birth control must be practiced for three months after the vaccine has been given so as not to expose a developing child to the effects of the vaccine.

If a pregnant woman is exposed to rubella, the following courses of action are available:

1. If it had been determined previously that the woman had immunity against rubella (by the blood test referred to above), there is no cause for concern.

2. If it had been determined that immunity did not exist at the beginning of pregnancy, further blood tests must be done to determine if in fact the woman in question was truly exposed. As mentioned above, one cannot rely on symptoms to determine if actual exposure occurred. Furthermore, rubella is sometimes difficult to diagnose and the suspected exposure may have been something other than rubella. If it is determined by blood tests that exposure occurred, then the possibility of therapeutic abortion can be presented —depending on the total medical, social, and religious situation of the patient.

3. If no previous determination of rubella immunity had occurred, the pregnant woman who has been possibly exposed should have a blood test done *immediately* when the possibility of exposure is determined. That immediate blood test followed by other blood tests will tell whether exposure occurred; if it did, the possibility of abortion can be considered.

The best approach is to make sure any woman of child-bearing age is immune (a blood test will tell) and to give the rubella vaccine (according to the precautions listed above) if the woman is not immune.

Headaches

Headaches are a real "headache" for both patient and doctor. For the patient, a headache means annoying pain and worry about "something serious" causing the headache. For the doctor a headache also means worry about the remote possibility of something serious—a tumor, meningitis, bleeding inside the skull, etc.

Fortunately, the vast majority of headaches are not life-threatening, either immediately or long-range. Those that are immediately life-threatening are almost invariably accompanied by other signs or symptoms: change in vision, speech or facial problems, loss of or decrease in the state of consciousness, etc. Any headache that is accompanied by such symptoms or that is extremely *sudden* and *severe* in onset ("like a bolt of lightning") must be investigated immediately at the nearest medical facility or emergency room.

But, as stated initially, most headaches are not emergencies. Indeed, most headaches are so-called "tension" headaches—caused by real tension (spasm) of the muscles of the head and neck and often related to emotional tension. Such headaches are most commonly located in the back of the head and/or over the eyes, but they may be felt anywhere and described in terms other than pain—dull, pressing, burning, etc. Applying gentle heat and/or massaging the neck muscles are usually very effective in relieving both the muscular and emotional tension. Ordinary aspirin should be sufficient if medicine is needed. If such headaches are associated with a fever or do not clear with this approach in twenty-four hours (or get progressively worse during such treatment), a call to your primary care physician is in order.

We are now left with two other headaches which deserve special mention since they are often difficult to diagnose and treat.

1. *Migraine headaches.* The keys to successful treatment of this type of headache are proper diagnosis followed by appropriate drug therapy. Proper diagnosis is easy in the classical cases—busy people with a family history of such headaches who are also perfectionistic and rigid, attacks which are preceded by sometimes strange mental, visual, or gastrointestinal symptoms, headaches which are described as throbbing in character and which are often one-sided, etc. However, headache experts are pointing out that migraine is more commonly "atypical" than we have previously suspected and that many unusual headache patterns turn out to be responsive to typical migraine therapy. Successful migraine therapy is based on the use of *appropriate* drugs *early* in the attack; a migraine headache is much easier to abort in the early stages than to treat when well established. The drug methysergide has been widely used to *prevent* migraines, but it is a potentially dangerous drug and must be taken only under the careful supervision of a physician familiar with the drug. More recently, propanalol has been successfully used in a preventive fashion. Almost all headache experts feel that attention to details of emotional and psychological concerns are essential in both prevention and treatment of migraine attacks.

2. *Cluster headaches.* These headaches are sometimes referred to as "Horton's" or "histamine" headaches because they were first described by Horton as related to histamine (a chemical found in our bodies). Such head-

aches are characterized by sudden onset of severe, one-sided pain usually accompanied by eye redness, tearing, and nasal stuffiness on the side of the pain; onset during sleep is common, but they can occur during the day. Although Horton originally recommended "desensitization" to histamine, these headaches are now considered to be a variant of migraine headaches and are treated as such. Since the natural history of such headaches is one of a series of brief attacks (clusters) separated by long periods without headaches, treatment is difficult to evaluate.

The above descriptions bring us to the most important issue to talk about in relation to problem headaches: What kind of doctor is best qualified to treat persistent problem headaches, and what kinds of tests are necessary to properly investigate such headaches? Persistent headaches should be initially seen by a competent primary care physician to rule out some of the general medical conditions which can cause headaches—anemia, hypertension, infections, etc. The following tests are often associated with a "headache workup" (in addition to a good history and physical):

A *skull X ray* should be done; while nothing is usually found, such X rays should be done since they are harmless and in rare cases pinpoint a serious problem. Also useful is a *blood count*—anemia and infection are worth checking for in all headaches. A *brain scan and EEG (electro-encephalogram)* are often ordered in problem headaches since they too are harmless and may demonstrate problems responsible for the headaches. (These tests are not to be confused with *cerebral angiography* or *pneumoencephalograms,* which are much more dangerous tests to be done under the direction of an appropriate specialist.) If there is any suspicion that a headache may be caused by infection and/or bleeding in the tissues of the brain or spinal cord, a *spinal tap* must be done to make such a diagnosis.

A spinal tap is not without danger, but done properly its risks are minimal compared to the risk of missing something which should be treated—such as meningitis.

Even after careful evaluation by a primary care physician some headaches will deserve the further attention of a specialist. In some large medical centers, certain physicians (usually either internists or neurologists) take a special interest in headaches and consequently become expert in diagnosing and often successfully treating headaches that have puzzled other physicians. Often this special interest means simply taking the time to do a thorough history and physical for clues that others might have missed. In the absence of such "headache specialists" the general neurologist is usually the physician most competent to diagnose and treat problem headaches; in some communities without a neurologist the neurosurgeon handles such problems.

Again I stress that a good primary care physician should be able to handle the majority of headaches. But, for those for whom headaches have become a major problem which interferes with normal living, the seeking out of a recognized headache authority may be worth the time and money required.

Hemorrhoids

These common and annoying veins of the anal area are important in two ways. First, in themselves they cause considerable discomfort and disability. And, second, they are often blamed for bleeding which may in fact be the result of other more serious problems—including colon and rectal cancer. For this reason, any treatment of hemorrhoids as a cause of bleeding must be preceded by barium enema and sigmoidoscopic examination to rule out other causes of the bleeding.

Appropriate treatment of hemorrhoids depends very much on individual circumstances—location, severity of symptoms, previous problems, etc. Most hemorrhoids can be treated conservatively, thus avoiding surgery. But in some cases, complete surgical removal of the hemorrhoids provides the best solution. A proctologist is a surgeon who specializes in these and other "end things" and is appropriate to consult. Most general surgeons are also competent in this area. One should be warned, however, that there are occasional doctors who run "hemorrhoid mills"—performing questionable procedures for high fees. Before any extensive therapy for hemorrhoids is performed you should do some checking with a good primary care physician.

Hyperactive Child

The hyperactive child bandwagon is an excellent example of an important medical advance in danger of excess application and enthusiasm. Make no mistake: The use of stimulant drugs for the treatment of the truly hyperactive child represents one of the great advances in pediatrics during the past twenty-five years. But there is now a clearly recognized danger that parents, teachers, and physicians might be too quick to apply the label "hyperactive" which usually leads automatically to drug therapy.

Hyperactivity implies excess motor activity (body movement). Actually, the syndrome is more properly described as activity which interferes with normal functioning at the given age level. For a two-year-old this might be the inability to "relax" enough to give or receive affection; a six-year-old might manifest difficulty by the inability to concentrate long enough to complete any school task. In other words, a diagnosis of hyperactivity requires careful and thorough evaluation—not just a casual observance of the physical activity of a child. Many experts suggest that hyperactivity is one manifestation of a larger condition called MBD—minimal brain damage; this phrase suggests that damage to the brain tissues too small to present as obvious physical or mental retardation might express itself in more subtle functional difficulties—such as hyperactivity. I personally find this concept of little use in dealing with lay people, since the phrase is often more frightening than illuminating. Hyperactivity does not imply brain damage, which dooms a person to an inferior life.

It is critical that a proper diagnosis be made of any child who manifests difficulty in living. Too often, hearing or vision problems are interpreted as psychological or hyperactive problems; the child who cannot sit still and pay attention may act that way because sensory stimuli are not getting through. Thus, before any label is placed on a child, a thorough physical and psychological screening is mandatory. Your pediatrician should be adequate to this task —and guide to referral sources as necessary.

Once an accurate diagnosis of hyperactivity has been established, treatment with stimulant drugs is the mainstay of therapy and is remarkably successful in most hyperactive children. Such successful treatment is marked by behavioral improvement in general and learning in particular. Some children are so sensitive to stimulant drugs that teachers and parents can tell if a single dose is missed. It seems strange that stimulant drugs should help a condition already marked by too much activity; such a drug reaction represents another example of the fact that drugs in children sometimes act opposite to the way they work in adults. Children should *not* be treated for hyperactivity with tranquilizing type drugs.

To date, the use of stimulant drugs in children appears relatively safe. I say "relatively" because one would prefer, in general, not to use drugs at all and because occasional reports of side effects do appear in the literature. One of the more serious of these reports appeared several years ago, suggesting that such drugs might produce growth retardation in children; however, no further substantiation has occurred and other investigators have not demonstrated this. You should certainly discuss the relative risks of the use of these drugs in your child in a frank and thorough way with your physician. Since they are so widely used (though not nearly as extensively as some alarmists have suggested), any clear danger from their use would become rapidly known and disseminated.

Finally, a word about therapy other than drugs. While drugs usually are the most important part of the treatment of the hyperactive child, total school and home approach is significant. For example, a hyperactive child may require different limits and goals than a child without such difficulty; this will obviously require special understanding by both parents and school officials. Both parents and physicians have a responsibility to see that all who deal with a hyperactive child are "clued in" to the best ways to help such a child.

Hypertension (*High Blood Pressure*)

More attention is being paid to this disease (in terms of public education) than any other because it has become clear in recent years that it pays—in terms of both lengthened life and improved life quality—to treat hypertension, including forms that were once considered too mild to need treatment. Too, there are millions of Americans who are hypertensive but are either undiagnosed or improperly treated.

That's the problem in a nutshell; here are some details.

Diagnosis

There continues to be some disagreement as to what blood pressure readings justify diagnosing a person as having "high" blood pressure. It is important to understand that a single blood pressure reading taken under conditions of concern (like a doctor's office visit) does not justify the label. It is just as important to understand that such a reading cannot be dismissed as being due to "the circumstances." In other words, a diagnosis of hypertension—which makes treatment mandatory—must be made with careful determinations over a period of time in more or less "normal" circumstances. (The exception to this, of course, is even a single reading that is "sky-high" and clearly abnormal.) If there is any question about a single reading, such a process of careful determination must be pursued. In the past, both doctors and patients have been too casual about making sure; if your doctor still is, then you must take charge and get your pressure checked—by anyone who can take a pressure reading.

The actual numbers that determine whether hypertension exists will vary with *age* (the older, the higher the numbers allowed), *sex* (at any age, males are more affected by high blood pressure than women), *race* (Black people are at greater risk from hypertension), and evidence of already existing *complications* from hypertension. For years the insurance companies have used 140/90 (one-forty over ninety) as a cutoff point; generally that's a good rule of thumb, but every case must be looked at individually.

A quick word about the numbers. The first number is

the *systolic* pressure, the second the *diastolic* pressure. The systolic pressure is that maximum pressure that occurs when the heart contracts and forces blood out through the arterial system under top pressure. The diastolic pressure is that minimum pressure that occurs in between heart contractions and therefore represents the constant pressure to which the arterial system is subjected. Since the diastolic pressure exists most of the time, it was felt for years that it was the most important pressure—i.e., the second number was more important than the first. That still is the general opinion, but it is now clear that the first number (the systolic pressure) is also very important and merits treatment when elevated abnormally.

Finally, in this section on diagnosis, a word of encouragement to anyone wishing to check their own pressures. The taking of blood pressures is a simple task given proper equipment, training, and experience. If there is reason for you to check your own pressures regularly, you should consider investment in your own equipment—a reasonably good stethoscope and blood pressure cuff-gauge (called a sphygmomanometer).

Why Get So Excited?

Reasonable question. And, in the shortest possible form, the answer: Untreated hypertension leads to a higher incidence of strokes, heart disease, and kidney failure. And those are bad diseases which can lead to untimely death.

In more detail: High blood pressure does a job on the arterial side of circulation leading to increased atherosclerosis (plugging by fatty material) and damage to those arteries. Doctors look in the back of the eye when diagnosing high blood pressure; the back of the eye is the one place where the arteries of our body are visible, and they tend to reflect the state of our arteries elsewhere.) This damage is particularly important in three organs, resulting in the following problems:

Heart: People with untreated high blood pressure have a higher incidence of heart attacks and heart failure. This is due to the fact that both atherosclerosis of the coronary arteries and weakening of the heart muscle are accelerated.

Brain: The arteries bringing blood to the brain are affected leading to a higher incidence of CVA's (cerebrovascular accidents or "strokes").

Kidneys: The arteries of the kidneys are affected, leading to permanent kidney damage and failure.

Treatment

It should now be obvious why we treat hypertension. What we are really doing is trying to prevent the damage hypertension can cause in our vital organs. In all honesty I cannot tell you that effective treatment will prevent all complications and correspondingly lengthen life. But it is now clear (from extensive studies on men in Veterans' hospitals) that treating even moderate elevations pays off more than enough to make it worthwhile.

Eighty-five percent of cases of high blood pressure turn out (after careful investigation) to have no clear cause and are therefore termed "essential hypertension." This unfortunate term stems from the days when hypertension was so commonly found that it was felt to be "essential" to the body. The remaining fifteen percent will be found to have some underlying disease (such as diseases of the adrenal gland) or a possibly surgically correctable abnormality (such as some narrowed arteries leading to the kidney).

For those with essential hypertension, treatment is loss of weight, a low-salt diet, and the careful selection and use of drugs. For some, weight loss and/or diet will be all that is required. A quick word of warning: Salt is everywhere in our diet and often hidden from view. When a low-salt diet is in order, very careful attention to hidden sources is required; diet charts are available to list such sources. Most persons with hypertension will require one or more of the many drugs now available. Drug therapy is both an art and a science in finding the best therapy with the least number of side effects. A good internist is the keynote to such therapy.

Surveys indicate that millions of people who should be treated are either undiagnosed or improperly treated. Many persons do not take medications as prescribed "because I feel so good." The point must be made that most hypertensive patients have no symptoms until the end stage of damage to the brain, heart, or kidneys. The idea that headaches or dizziness accompanies hypertension is so only for a small number; *most have no symptoms.*

So we are back where we started. The story of hypertension begins with careful attention to diagnosis, which means getting your blood pressure checked whenever and wherever possible. This is one case when a good cuff on the arm might pay off.

Hypoglycemia

This word means, literally, "low blood sugar." Unfortunately, the word is also, in our present society, a rallying point for people with many of the vague symptoms that afflict modern man—fatigue, listlessness, headaches, jitteriness, etc. And, doubly unfortunately, there are physicians who foster the fad of hypoglycemia for financial gain.

Almost everyone has "low blood sugar" at some time

during the day; an isolated blood test demonstrating a lower than usual blood sugar is not synonymous with a diagnosis of hypoglycemia. The diagnosis of true hypoglycemia (as a disease) requires the demonstration of the following three components:

1. The careful demonstration of low blood sugar in a glucose tolerance test—which requires the drinking of a heavy sugar solution and up to six hours of serial blood samples, drawn at half-hourly to hourly intervals

2. The appearance of symptoms *simultaneously* with low blood sugars

3. The almost immediate relief of symptoms with the administration of intravenous glucose

The most important task facing the physician who suspects hypoglycemia is to distinguish between "organic" and "functional" hypoglycemia. Organic hypoglycemia is very rare and is caused by a variety of diseases and tumors which act to cause imbalance in the delicate mechanisms by which the body keeps the blood sugar in a normal range. (The crucial reason for keeping the blood sugar in a normal range is that the brain is extremely dependent on sugar for its functioning and the brain will not function properly when sugar is low; in extreme states of low blood sugar, coma and death can result.)

Functional hypoglycemia (also called "reactive," "spontaneous," "neurogenic") is much more common but less well understood. In most cases, this type of hypoglycemia is thought to be due to insulin excess (which will lower blood sugar), but that cannot always be demonstrated. Generally this type of hypoglycemia is treated by diet modifications, which include more frequent but smaller feedings low in sugar. While this seems like strange treatment for low blood sugar, the theory is that, if the problem is overreaction to ingested sugar by the body's control mechanism, keeping the sugar content of our food low will prevent this overreaction. In most cases, this approach seems to work.

Obviously this subject is complex and requires the skills of a good primary care physician and often the help of an endocrinologist. And I return to my original points: Hypoglycemia is rare and cannot be diagnosed casually on the basis of a single blood test. There is a strong psychological component in many of the symptoms that have been tied to hypoglycemia, and these symptoms may therefore respond to sympathy and shots of sugar water. I have no quarrel with this as long as people can afford such treatment and no harm is being done. But when such "treatments" cover up curable problems or miss organic disease they border on malpractice.

If you have read much of this book you know by now that I seldom quote "official" medical organizations for support. However, the subject of hypoglycemia is so laden with emotion that I deem it appropriate to quote the following material from an official statement cosponsored by the American Diabetes Association, the Endocrine Society, and the American Medical Association:

Hypoglycemia means a low level of blood sugar. When it occurs, it is often attended by symptoms of sweating, shakiness, trembling, anxiety, fast heart action, headache, hunger sensations, brief feelings of weakness, and, occasionally, seizures and coma. However, the majority of people with these kinds of symptoms do not have hypoglycemia; a great many patients with anxiety reactions present with similar symptoms. Furthermore, there is no good evidence that hypoglycemia causes depression, chronic fatigue, allergies, nervous breakdowns, alcoholism, juvenile delinquency, childhood behavior problems, drug addiction or inadequate sexual performance. There are many causes of hypoglycemia. . . . Treatment depends on which pattern is observed and on the particular cause of the hypoglycemia which exists. . . . There is no place for injections in the treatment of the common reactive types of low blood sugar . . . it should be stressed that administration of adrenal cortical extract is not an appropriate treatment for any cause of hypoglycemia.

Immunizations

There is increasing alarm among public health officials concerning the growing lack of concern about immunizations. Control of infectious disease is taken for granted in generations removed from the days of polio epidemics. The fact is that there is *no more important* or effective health measure than careful attention to full immunization. The currently recommended schedule is as follows:

Recommended Schedule for Active Immunization of Children

AGE	PRODUCT ADMINISTERED
2–3 months	DTP (diphtheria/tetanus/pertussis)
	Oral polio vaccine, trivalent
3–4 months	DTP
	Oral polio vaccine, trivalent
4–5 months	DTP
	Oral polio vaccine, trivalent
12–14 months	Measles-mumps-rubella vaccines (either singly or in combination)
	DTP
	Oral polio vaccine, trivalent
6 years	TD
	Oral polio vaccine, trivalent
12–14 years	TD

Several comments are now in order:

1. *Smallpox* vaccination is no longer recommended as a routine procedure. We have now reached the point in this country (and most of the world) where the risk of reactions from the vaccination is greater than the risk of getting the disease. Smallpox vaccination is still legitimate for persons traveling to areas of high risk.

2. *Polio* vaccination is *a must!* Oral trivalent (meaning three types in a combined dose) is the best, though the Salk (inactive, injected) is still available. Note that three doses are given in the first year and then a booster about a year later. There is great concern on the part of public health officials that we may be facing a serious polio epidemic since so many children are not receiving routine immunizations.

3. *Measles* vaccine is one of the newer ones. Most people are not aware of the very serious complications (often leading to death) that can occur with measles; fortunately they are rare, but the risk is there and the vaccine should be used. There are several different types of vaccine; some are best given with a gamma-globulin shot in the other arm to minimize reaction.

4. *Rubella* (German measles) vaccination has been controversial from the start. The controversy is not about the safety (except for pregnant women) or effectiveness of the vaccine but only about when it should be used and how long its effects will last. Specifically, some propose mass immunization in childhood as suggested in the schedule above. Others propose that it should be given selectively only to those women entering puberty who have not developed natural immunity. (Remember that the disease—unlike regular

measles—is not dangerous to the person getting it but to the developing fetus of the pregnant women who gets it.) Since this controversy is between experts, I do not propose to settle it. Most experts favor the mass immunization approach and recent evidence tends to support this in terms of the lasting effect of the vaccine. Again I stress that the vaccine should not be given to any adult woman in whom there is a chance of pregnancy or in whom pregnancy is anticipated in the near future (within three months). (See German measles.)

5. *Tuberculosis* testing (not listed) is often neglected as part of routine childhood health care; that is a big mistake—it should be done. The actual frequency of testing will depend on the risk of exposure for the given child. (See Tuberculosis.)

6. *Tetanus* is still a danger—especially to those who missed basic childhood immunizations, such as the elderly of our society. Tetanus is the T of the DTP in the schedule; by schooltime, pertussis (P)—whooping cough—should no longer be included in vaccine preparations.

Finally, another reminder to keep accurate immunization records at home. When you need them, the doctor's office or hospital record room is invariably closed.

Infertility

The usual definition of infertility is the absence of conception after one year of normal sexual relations without contraception between a given couple. Approximately ten percent of marriages in this country are infertile by this standard. In those cases studied, about sixty percent of the causes can be traced to the female partner, forty percent to the male. Apart from any specific problem in either partner, the chances of conception are related to four factors: (1) age of the female partner (maximal around age twenty-four and much less after age thirty); (2) age of male partner (about the same—much less after age forty); (3) frequency of intercourse (four times per week is ideal for conception); and (4) length of relationship (sixty-three percent of couples will conceive in six months, ninety percent in eighteen months).

So much for statistics. For any given couple, statistics do not help. Diagnosis and treatment must be given individually and must include careful consideration of the emotional environment involved. Obviously, the personality of the physician to whom the couple turns can be very important; this is one of the more important choices to be made in medical care. Two specialists are usually involved in infertility problems—the gynecologist and the urologist. Generally, the gynecologist will direct the entire effort and call in the urologist as needed. Not all gynecologists are competent to handle complex infertility problems, either the physical or the emotional component. In any given community, there are usually several gynecologists who have become identified as experts in infertility problems. You should seek them out in any manner possible; Planned Parenthood is sometimes a good source of advice.

It would not serve any useful purpose in this book to list all the possible causes of infertility in both partners; they range from anatomical problems which might be surgically correctable to hormonal imbalances which might be responsive to medication. It is useful, however, to stress that any success in diagnosis and treatment depends on the cooperation of both husband and wife. Too often, the male either openly or passively blames the female for the absence of conception; the figures cited earlier indicate a significant male factor.

I would like to comment on two drugs used in infertility treatment, since they are often confused and this confusion may even prevent couples from seeking help. Both drugs are used to stimulate ovulation—the release of the egg from the ovary of the female. First is *Clomiphene (Clomid)*. This drug has been extensively used in the past decade. Its mechanism of action involves stimulation of a certain area of the brain which releases "messengers" which in turn stimulate the release of the hormones which cause ovulation (release of the egg). Multiple pregnancies —almost always twins—occur in about one of sixteen pregnancies achieved with Clomid (versus one of eighty in the general population).

Second is *human menopausal gonadotropin (HMG— Pergonal)*. This drug is obtained from the urine of postmenopausal women. The incidence of multiple pregnancies with this drug is high—about one of five. Most of these multiple pregnancies are twins (eighty percent), but *this* is the "fertility drug" that causes the large multiple births you often read about. It should be stressed that Clomid is the more commonly used drug, so that you should not be put off by the possibility of large multiple births. Pergonal is used only after careful consultation between you and your physician; you obviously do not have to agree to its use. Most gynecologists refer patients needing Pergonal to infertility specialists or to university centers.

Finally, a brief note about artificial insemination. Using the husband's sperm, the procedure has not been very successful. Using a donor's sperm, the procedure is quite successful. The decision to use this procedure—and especially a donor's sperm—obviously requires mature and careful consideration by the couple.

I will close this section by again urging that couples interested in seeking help for conception spend time and effort in seeking the appropriate physician—one who is knowledgeable and supportive. This kind of "infertility doctor" does not grow on every corner.

Obesity

Though I am tempted to do otherwise, I will limit this section to a discussion of the relationship between obesity and health. (The temptation lies in the direction of commentary about the social and moral implications of obesity as a major problem in a world where starvation daily claims the lives of thousands of people.) I have relied heavily on an excellent summary by Dr. George Mann in the July 25, and August 1, 1974, issues of the *New England Journal of Medicine,* "The Influence of Obesity on Health."

As Dr. Mann points out, the question of the relationship of obesity to health is not an insignificant one, since many industries—from life insurance to those involved with weight control—have profited from the general fear of fatness. Apart from the question of the physical health hazards posed by obesity, few would disagree that obesity produces psychological ill-being, which is reason enough to consider weight reduction to be a legitimate health activity. But that belief is no excuse for inaccurate information regarding health and obesity.

One of the questions posed by experts on "body fat" is how to accurately measure excess body fat. ("Bigness" is not synonymous with "fatness.") And, while this question is important for the research efforts of experts, I would suggest that for most of us the question represents an effort to avoid the truth. I am reminded of the comment made by an expert on the subject after a day-long discussion of how best to determine obesity. He suggested that the subject in question (you and I) take off all clothes, stand in front of a full length mirror, and turn around slowly. At that point it boils down to the fact that, "if you look fat, you are fat."

The information on obesity is itself massive. I may be oversimplifying, but I would like to summarize what I think is most important about the subject by answering the following questions:

Is Fatness Caused by Something Wrong in the Body Metabolism?

In only a *very rare* instance is this true. The vast majority of weight problems are due to excess calories consumed in relationship to physical activity.

As is the case with alcoholism, there has been an intensive research effort to find a "missing enzyme" (or some similar biochemical defect) which would not only give fatness respectability but, more important, provide the possibility of "medical" cure. And, while much suggestive animal research has been reported, there is no firm evidence in humans.

Another approach has been to suggest a genetic component. Most authorities would recognize a genetic role in that net result we label obesity, but, whatever that role, it has been greatly overshadowed by "environment"— i.e., caloric input and life-style.

Are There "Critical Periods" for the Development of Fat Cells?

During the past five years, a theory has been developed by several researchers to suggest that a person who develops obesity in childhood has two strikes against him (or her) because such a person develops excess fat cells early in life resulting in a lifelong struggle to keep those extra fat cells "slimmed down." This theory is intuitively attractive and jibes with the experience of many people for whom "dieting" is a constant necessity in relation to their appetite desires.

Some researchers, including Mann, doubt the validity of this theory; such critics point out the great difficulty of accurately measuring numbers of fat cells. There is, however, considerable agreement among obesity experts that patterns of eating and exercise established in childhood have a profound effect on later life habits. It is also now apparent that children must be "taught" (not necessarily in a verbal way) how to "use food properly"; if left to their own devices entirely, they will not make proper dietary choices.

Is Obesity Dangerous to Health?

We have all been brought up on the idea that the answer to this question is yes. It is constantly pointed out that "you don't see many fat old people walking around." Most doctors and insurance companies reinforce this idea by word (the lecture) and deed (no insurance, higher premiums).

The hard facts are that obesity is not a major physical health hazard when compared, for example, to smoking. Notice that I have inserted the word physical because it is obvious that most people "feel" better—about the world and themselves—when not overweight. And the longer I live, the more impressed I am with the value of psychic health. So I am not saying that obesity is good. But honesty compels me to say that we are not as sure about the physical health hazards as we have led most people to believe. Let's be more specific.

Coronary heart disease: The contribution of obesity to this disease is extremely small. One of the "ideas" ingrained in our medical mentalities is that obesity causes a mechanical strain on our hearts. There is no evidence to support that and one might well conjecture the opposite —that extra weight "exercises" the heart in a salutory fashion. (Sorry; no evidence for that either.)

This is a good place to put one other myth to rest. Many people say they can't stop smoking because if they do they will gain weight, which poses a health hazard. There is no question that most people put on weight when they stop smoking. But there is no comparison between the health effects of smoking (twenty-three times greater chance of lung cancer, two to three times greater chance of heart attack) and excess weight. From a health standpoint, excess weight for no cigarettes is an excellent trade.

Hypertension: First, it should be emphasized that blood pressure readings will be falsely elevated if the bladder of the cuff used to encircle the arm does not also encircle the arm. But, given this common error, there is no doubt that high blood pressure is more common among obese people and that high blood pressure is a potent risk factor for coronary heart disease. Studies have shown that persons twenty percent or more overweight had a ten times greater chance of developing high blood pressure, and we know that sustained high blood pressure does affect the arteries of the brain, heart, and kidney, causing serious disease. (See Hypertension.)

Pregnancy: This subject is treated more fully in the section on *Obstetrical Care.* Suffice it to say at this point that the past emphasis on minimal weight gain during pregnancy was ill-advised at best and dangerous at worst.

We now know that good maternal nutrition is vital to healthy development of the unborn baby and that the optimal weight gain during pregnancy for Western women is about twenty-four to twenty-seven pounds (assuming that gain represents sound nutrition), including a gain of about one pound per week during the second half of pregnancy. It is also worth pointing out here that breast feeding is ideal for both restoring energy balance in the mother and minimizing obesity in the newborn; commercial milk formulas tend to overfeed babies.

Diabetes: It is well known that adult-onset diabetes is more common among the obese and that weight control is a useful part of treatment in such people. Whether obesity per se is a cause of diabetes is less clear.

Again I stress that the above information is not intended to support obesity. It is merely to summarize in an honest way what we know about health hazards of fatness. Since the psychological value of proper weight is sufficient reason for such pursuit, let's turn to the evaluation of treatment possibilities.

What Treatment(s) Are the Most Successful for Obesity?

In a word, none are spectacular but approaches combining group therapy and behavior modification are clearly the most effective. TOPS (Take Off Pounds Sensibly) is a non-profit organization (as opposed to Weight Watchers) which has demonstrated average weight losses of fifteen pounds persisting for sixteen or more months. A word about other treatment approaches is in order:

Drugs: I personally would like to see appetite suppressant drugs taken off the market. Most physicians do not share that opinion. There is no question that such drugs can be useful for short-term appetite suppression; indeed, they can be so used hundreds of times—which is the problem. Apart from their lack of effectiveness, such drugs present the real problem of drug abuse. There is no role for thyroid drugs. The effectiveness of "gonadotropins" (hormone injections) is not established.

Diets: Diets alone rarely work—except to make money for the promoter and book writer. When *any* diet does work it is because less calories are consumed. It has been demonstrated that diets that promise "you can eat as much as you want" of something work because after a while that "something" becomes sickening so you eat less. The Atkins diet is not only based on questionable theory, but its long-term effects (stressing fat consumption) could be injurious to the cardiovascular system. Total fasts should be done only under medical supervision.

Ileal Bypass Surgery: This major surgery (which diverts food past much of the absorptive area of the small intestine) should be reserved for the severely obese for whom all other approaches to weight loss have failed. The surgery is dangerous both in the immediate operative period and in the long-term effects on the liver. Such surgery should be done only in centers where careful selection and post-operative supervision is available.

Hypnosis: There are no good studies yet to demonstrate the effectiveness of this approach. Too often it is offered at outrageous prices. However, I am impressed with anecdotal "evidence" about hypnosis as a tool for both weight loss and smoking abstinence. It may turn out to be useful if done at a reasonable cost by appropriately trained people.

Exercise: As mentioned in the section on nutrition, exercise has considerable psychological value for many people, but losing weight is not one of the more prominent results of casual exercise. Studies show that *regular* exercise contributes to appropriate weight, apparently more by appetite regulation than calorie consumption. The most impressive result of exercise to me, as a physician, has been the number of sore feet and sprained joints in persons who have jumped into an exercise regime without appropriate conditioning. Excessive exercise in a middle-aged person may be dangerous; a medical O.K. should be obtained first.

In Summary

Obesity has probably been overemphasized as a physical health hazard. For a doctor, the easiest way out is to "lay down the law" without considering the individual involved as a total person, not just an energy machine out of whack. There are, however, very legitimate health reasons for striving for a reasonably ideal weight. The best approach seems to be a "group-therapy" approach where peer pressure aids the process of changing basic eating habits.

Obstetrical Care

The title of this section is chosen to convey the fact that the selectivity involved is that of attempting to discuss "what's new" in obstetrics. It would be impossible to deal with the entirety of the emotional and physical experience we call pregnancy—impossible both because of the space limitations of this book *and* because of my personal limitations as a male physician. I recommend the book *Our Bodies, Ourselves,* by the Boston Women's Health Book Collective, which presents the view of knowledgeable lay women with strong emphases on both fact and opinion. So what I really propose to do in this section is summarize some of the more important information that every person related to the pregnancy experience (that includes us, men) should know about.

Before doing so, I must comment on the question of home versus hospital deliveries. Actually, the choice is not quite that stark—where home is defined as the bedroom with no expertise or equipment and hospital is defined as the obstetrical ward of a large impersonal hospital. There are middle ground alternatives—more developed in Europe than in this country—where equipment and personnel (usually well-trained midwives) can be brought to the home *or* where hospital settings are more homelike in attitude and layout. If the expertise and equipment are available to handle the small number of dangerous complications at delivery, then the actual setting becomes a matter of personal preference. The fact is that in this country such expertise and equipment can seldom be offered outside the hospital. But, where it can and the preference of the couple involved is for a home delivery, I think the medical profession should be receptive and not reject the idea just because of personal preference or bias. In other words, I can't answer the question of "home" versus "hospital" deliveries because there are so many variables involved in any given case. Honesty compels me to warn both of the very real complications that arise in about 5 percent of deliveries *and* of the bias of most physicians against even reasonable alternatives to the traditional obstetrical ward atmosphere.

Which leads me to the changes that are occurring in many obstetrical wards—fathers in the delivery room, babies staying with mothers (so-called "rooming in"), concern with the psyche as well as the physical needs of the mother, etc. "Family-centered" maternity care is a phrase now being used to describe an obstetrical ward which attempts to meet the needs of the mother and new family on an individual basis—not forcing the baby on the mother when she doesn't want the responsibility but making the baby available when she does; also implied in this concept is a large amount of teaching to aid the mother and father in adjusting to their new responsibility. I am for these changes 100 percent; there is no doubt in my mind that the male dominance of obstetrics has hindered these changes from occurring since there is no sound medical data to suggest any harm from them. The only word of caution I would offer is that an equally rigid attitude in the opposite direction should not force parents into accepting some of these new ideas and routines if they do not wish them.

Two final opinions are in order. First, any hospital which does less than 1500 deliveries per year may be inadequate to handle the emergencies and complications of delivery. I say "may" because there will be exceptions—and the mere fact of 1500 or more deliveries per year does not guarantee adequate obstetrical care. This number of 1500 has been proposed by the American College of Obstetrics and Gynecologists. Second, the role of the GP in obstetrics is rapidly being restricted to routine prenatal care—if even that. Again, there will be exceptions; but, in general, a GP doing only occasional deliveries is no match for the daily experience of a fully trained obstetrician.

Now, on to the more medical considerations relating to pregnancy.

Prepared (Natural) Childbirth

I start off with this subject because it still is rife with opinion and controversy. The traditional approach of the medical profession has been that of rather routinely medicating the woman in labor to minimize pain and memory; scopolomine is the drug most commonly used to effect the latter—i.e., to cause the patient to forget any pain or unpleasantness related to the delivery. Many other medications may be used during the labor process. And at the time of actual delivery, other medications plus general anesthesia may be used.

"Prepared" childbirth means just what is said—being prepared for the experience of childbirth. It does not mean painless childbirth. It does not mean natural childbirth in the sense that nothing can or should be done to modify the course of pregnancy or delivery. It *does* mean that being physically *and* mentally prepared for childbirth will decrease the fear and pain traditionally associated with the experience. It suggests that the woman so prepared will be less likely to need drugs and will be more likely to be able to experience childbirth as an involved participant rather than a zonked-out and passive "deliverer" of this child she has nurtured for nine months. Such preparation involves work and thought, but I have observed that the effort is almost always well worth the result.

The details of such preparation are beyond the scope of this book. The Boston Women's Health Collective book discusses the subject in great detail and provides a good bibliography. My point here is to give the subject medical respectability and to urge anyone contemplating pregnancy and/or preparing for delivery to study the concepts and details of prepared childbirth.

Prenatal Care—High-Risk Pregnancy

Even though the mortality rates of pregnancy for both mother and child have been significantly reduced during the past forty years, far too many unnecessary (potentially preventable) deaths still occur. Most of these deaths could be prevented by better prenatal care—which implies responsibility for both physician and patient.

One of the concepts that has emerged from improved

obstetrical care is that of the "high-risk" pregnancy—i.e., those pregnancies which can be identified as being more likely to involve difficulty for mother and/or child and which should therefore be followed with even greater than usual care. The following are included in this category of higher risk:

1. *Any history of:*
   Hereditary abnormality (such as mongolism)
   Premature or small-for-dates delivery or unexplained fetal death
   Medical problems associated with previous pregnancy (toxemia, etc.)
   Prolonged infertility
   General medical or specific female medical problems

2. *Present pregnancy involving:*
   High-risk social conditions such as teenage mother, drug addiction, etc.
   Heavy cigarette smoking
   Long-delayed or absent prenatal care
   Possible damage from exposure to drugs, irradiation, illness, etc.
   Previous delivery within two months of current pregnancy
   Age greater than thirty-five
   Four or more previous deliveries

3. *Diagnosis or development of:*
   Height of mother under sixty inches or prepregnant weight greatly under or over the standard for height and age
   Minimal or no weight gain (or weight loss)
   Obstetrical complications (toxemia, multiple pregnancy, Rh disease, bleeding, etc.)
   Abnormal presentation (breech, etc.)

The point is that such factors mean that the pregnancy must be monitored with great diligence and care—including the use of amniocentesis, X ray (when essential), etc.

Nutrition

Most physicians and pregnant women have gotten the word that weight restriction is not nearly as important as it was thought to be. In fact, it may be dangerous. It is now clearly recognized that good nutrition is one of the most important keys to a healthy pregnancy. The praise for the woman who stays slim throughout her pregnancy ("I didn't even know she was pregnant") may be falsely placed. In other words, weight gain is an insensitive measure of nutritional status. It is possible to be slim, but in good nutritional "shape"—or to gain a large amount of weight and still be undernourished.

Thus, the actual weight gain that is optimal will vary for each woman. Here I wish only to stress the following:

1. Good nutrition even before starting a pregnancy is helpful. This is one of the problems, generally, with teenage pregnancies.

2. Pregnancy is no time to start dieting. Excess weight will have to be dealt with *after* pregnancy, but dieting which limits required nutrients during pregnancy deprives the developing fetus.

3. The last three months require the most increase in nutrients for the developing fetus. If a pregnant woman approaches these last months with a weight gain already greater than proposed for her entire pregnancy, she should not start dieting in order to attempt to meet her quota for the entire pregnancy.

There is much we still do not know about nutrition during pregnancy. It is, however, clear that poor nutrition and restricted maternal weight gain result in a greater chance of an unhealthy baby. This is a subject that you should discuss frankly and thoroughly during your first visit with your obstetrician.

P.S. While the exact role of iron, calcium, and folic acid supplements during pregnancy is not known, most experts agree they should be taken.

The First Three Months

While all of pregnancy should be treated with respect in terms of the potential danger of drugs and other "foreign" materials (irradiation, smoking), the first three months are particularly critical; it is during these months that the developing child completes the most critical phases of its development and it is during this time, therefore, that the most damage can be done.

The rule, of course, is that *no* medications should be taken by the pregnant woman without first checking with her doctor. Even an apparently innocuous medicine— such as aspirin—may be dangerous. Always check. Part of the problem is that medicines (or radiation) may be given to a woman *before* she knows she is pregnant. Doctors should know enough to check on the possibility of pregnancy before giving potentially dangerous medicines or ordering potentially damaging tests. But doctors forget or are not as sensitive as they should be. So *you* better be prepared to protect your own bodies.

Recently there has been some renewed concern about birth control pills causing deformed children. It should be made clear that this concern arises only if the pill (or other forms of hormone treatment) is taken *when* the woman is pregnant. This can occur if a woman starts the pill without first making sure she is not pregnant or if the woman takes the pill irregularly and becomes pregnant during this irregular pill usage. Another danger is posed by the use of hormonal tests of pregnancy—i.e., giving hormones to see if menstrual bleeding will occur. Such tests should no longer be used, especially since better non-hormonal tests are now readily available.

Amniocentesis

This subject is discussed in the section on genetic counseling, but I wish also to mention it as a part of this discussion and to stress its increasing value in diagnosing conditions which *may* influence a given couple to consider abortion as an alternative to the birth of a defective child. The major point I wish to make here is that of the timing involved. Amniocentesis cannot be done until about the fourteenth week of pregnancy; it then takes another two weeks to study the fluid and cells obtained by the procedure. In other words, if abortion is to be considered because of possible medical problems, prenatal care and amniocentesis must be sought *early* in the pregnancy.

Many experts are now saying that any pregnant woman over thirty-five (some would place the limit at forty) should have amniocentesis since the risk of abnormalities in general and Down's syndrome (mongolism) in particular is much greater in the pregnancy of an older woman.

Fetal Monitoring and Care

One of the most significant advances in obstetrical care during the past ten years has been the development of the knowledge and hardware to monitor the health of the fetus during the period of labor and delivery. Such monitoring involves attaching "wires" to the abdomen of the mother and/or the scalp of the child (via the mother's birth canal). While such monitoring is becoming routine in many hospitals, it should at least be mandatory in any high-risk delivery or when a problem develops during labor or delivery. So ask about such monitoring when you are choosing an obstetrician.

Breast Feeding

There is an old axiom that says "breast feeding is the best feeding." From a strictly medical view, that is sound advice. All else being close to equal, breast feeding offers both physical and psychological nurture which usually cannot be matched by bottle feeding. And not to be ignored are the secondary benefits of cost and convenience.

However, I stop short of the rigid philosophy which says that mothers must breast feed and that those who do not are less than adequate mothers. There are many sound reasons why some women should not breast feed, and I include among them the right of the woman to choose not to do so for reasons of personal convenience. From a medical viewpoint, bottle feeding is certainly adequate and may at times be even medically necessary to meet special needs of the baby. And I remind you that it is now known that breast feeding does *not* protect against breast cancer.

But my original statement still stands: Breast feeding, all else being close to equal, offers superior physical and psychological nurture. And, too often the woman who desires to breast feed is discouraged by lack of support from family or doctor or lack of adequate information. The La Leche League book (*The Womanly Art of Breastfeeding*) offers a great amount of specific information which can be very useful if separated from the sometimes rigid philosophy of that organization.

In Summary

I have attempted only to highlight some of the newer concerns of the period we call pregnancy. No other experience of life—except death—is as personal or as intense, physiologically or psychologically. This uniqueness makes the choice of doctor and delivery site even more critical than usual. I have not attempted to deal with some of the psychological issues involved but I again recommend the appropriate sections of the Boston Women's Health Collective book (as described in the Bibliography)—both for its content and its suggestions for further information.

Pain

This subject must be approached in two ways in the context of this book—pain as a new symptom requiring investigation and pain as an established problem requiring relief.

Pain as a new symptom is treated much the same as fever; it may or may not be significant depending on the total situation. Obviously we have all experienced fleeting "pains" which have turned out to be unimportant and unexplained. On the other hand, pain does not have to be severe or even persistent to be ultimately significant. For example, the pain of a heart attack may be ignored as a stomach upset until it is too late. And, as pointed out about fever, pain may not be a reliable indicator of serious disease in the very young or very old. All of which is to say what was said at the beginning of this paragraph: Pain is simply one factor in the total picture and cannot be relied upon—either by its presence or absence—to signal serious disease. As a general rule, any pain that persists (more than a few hours) or is associated with other symptoms (difficulty breathing or prolonged constipation, etc.) should be checked. Pain is an important indicator of trouble and should not be ignored when severe or persistent or associated with other problems.

And the doctor should treat pain not as a disease but as a guide. This is why we often will not completely eliminate pain (though this is usually possible with the potent pain medicines available) until we are sure as to the cause of the pain; we sometimes have to sacrifice total comfort until we know what we are dealing with and can be sure it is safe to treat the pain vigorously. For example, abdominal pain is an important guide to what is going on inside the abdomen; the elimination of such pain may mask a developing disaster and removing a valuable warning sign as to what is going on.

Pain as an established problem presents a different challenge. I am talking now about pain whose cause has been established or for which no known reason can be found after exhaustive investigation—including, often, exploratory surgery to look for the cause. While this is not a common problem, it is, for the patient and doctor involved, one of the most difficult problems in medicine. It is beyond the scope of this book to discuss all the possibilities and problems involved in dealing with so-called "intractable pain" but I should point out that many major teaching hospitals and medical schools have now established "pain clinics" to deal with such problems; they would be worth investigating if you have such a problem.

Parkinson's Disease

The treatment of this disease certainly meets one of the criteria of selection for this book—namely, a significant development that everyone should know about. Actually, anyone directly concerned with this disease has undoubtedly gotten the message that the administration of L-dopa (which acts to increase certain chemicals thought to be deficient in Parkinson's disease) represents a very significant breakthrough in treatment. I would only add the following general comments about treatment of this not uncommon disease:

1. While L-dopa and some of its newer variants are a great breakthrough, they do not work in all cases. Indeed, as more experience with the drug accumulates, it has become clear that it will not be as widely applicable as was originally hoped. Side-effects may be very significant.

2. There are many other drugs (so-called anticholinergics and antihistamines) which are still very useful, often in addition to L-dopa. The individual administration of these drugs is an art that requires patience and experience; a neurologist is usually the most familiar with the use of these drugs.

3. While surgery is much less used since the development of good drug therapy, there is still a role for the newer technique of "stereotaxic" surgery (involving very precise destruction of very small parts of the brain). There is still controversy as to exactly which part of the brain should be so treated. Surgery is generally best for young patients in otherwise good health with predominant symptoms of one-sided tremor (shaking) and rigidity (muscle stiffness.)

One final note: Many persons are needlessly fearful that they have Parkinson's disease because they have a tremor or shaking of their head and/or limbs. This symptom in itself is not diagnostic of Parkinson's but is more indicative of a milder problem known as essential or benign tremor. Benign tremor does not respond to L-dopa but does respond to other medications.

Prostate Disease

First, a lesson in spelling. Notice that the word does *not* have two "r's" in it. You may fall prostrate on the ground but you do not have a gland by that name.

Now that you have become instantaneously sophisticated about how to spell and pronounce "prostate," we can move on. The prostate gland is located deep in the pelvis of the male at the base of the penis; it contributes secretions to the semen during ejaculation. Because it opens into the urethra, through which both urine and semen pass, the prostate gland sometimes communicates its abnormalities via urinary symptoms—frequency, painful urination, pus and blood in the urine, etc. Noninfectious disease of the prostate, however, may be difficult to diagnose except by direct touching and/or biopsy of the gland.

Prostatitis (Infection)

Infection of the prostate gland is very common. Acute infections act very much like urinary tract infections and are treated with appropriate antibiotics. The acutely infected gland is often very tender when the doctor tries to feel it during a rectal exam.

Much more troublesome is so-called "chronic prostatitis." There is considerable controversy as to just what causes this problem and whether or not it is a true infection. Germs not ordinarily responsive to antibiotics are being implicated in chronic prostatitis and this may explain why response to antibiotics in the past has not always been successful. Prostatic massage has sometimes been helpful in chronic cases.

Prostate Tumors

As always, it is important to distinguish between benign and malignant tumors. In the case of the prostate gland, it is especially important, since benign tumors are very common and may be confused with the less common but not unusual malignant tumors of the gland.

Benign enlargement of the gland is referred to as BPH —benign prostatic hypertrophy (or hyperplasia). BPH is almost a normal part of aging; most men over age sixty will have some enlargement of their prostate. Since the prostate gland encircles the urethra as it passes from the bladder out the penis, it does not take much imagination to envision the effects of such enlargement. And, indeed, these effects are so well known to the human race that they are summarized (by the medical profession) in a word—*prostatism:* difficulty starting and maintaining urination, reduced force of the urinary stream and increased frequency of urination at night (nocturia). Such a constellation of symptoms suggests an enlarged prostate.

We have now come to the point where I can stress that a rectal examination should be a part of every physical examination. Such an exam is important for many reasons (rectal tumors, hidden blood in the stool, etc.) *including* the opportunity to feel the posterior part of the prostate gland through the front wall of the rectum. (Now you should understand that, when the doctor turns his finger around and presses against the front of the rectum during a rectal exam, he is feeling for the prostate gland.)

If an enlarged gland is found, the question of cancer—versus BPH—must be raised. Sometimes the shape and consistency of the gland will offer good clues (cancer usually produces hard growth). But more often, a biopsy will be necessary to make the diagnosis. (A biopsy is always required before radical prostate surgery is performed.) Biopsies can be done in several ways (including tissue obtained with a needle), and the advice of a good urologist is essential.

Benign enlargement of the prostate gland can be handled with relatively simple surgical removal of part or all of the gland; the most common method (done under anesthesia) involves removal done by scraping the inner part of the prostate out through a tube inserted via the penis.

Cancer of the prostate requires more radical surgery; the entire gland plus some surrounding tissue must be removed before spread occurs to effect permanent cure. However, hormonal therapy of prostate cancer has also proven useful; this may be accomplished by both direct administration of female hormones and orchidectomy (removal of the testicles) to remove the major source of male hormones. All of this obviously suggests that management of prostate cancer is complex and requires the skills of both urological and cancer specialists.

Seizures

Seizure disorders (of which epilepsy is one) represent a very complex medical subject; diagnosis and treatment often require thoughtful attention to both the physical and emotional needs of the patient. The subject in its entirety is beyond the scope of this book, but I would like to single out certain points which everyone should be aware of.

Emergency Reaction to a Seizure

Most of us will be exposed to a person having a seizure at some time in our lives—though this becomes less of a possibility as good drug control is the rule rather than the exception. If you find yourself in the presence of someone having a seizure, you should remember that there is little you need to do except protect the person from injuring himself. If the seizure is extensive (so-called "grand mal") the person will usually fall to the floor or the ground. You should move nearby objects, loosen clothing around the neck, and, if possible, insert something firm (but not rock-hard) between the teeth. *Do not* put your fingers in the mouth of a person who is seizing; you will not be able to keep the mouth open and you are likely to lose a finger. Usually the seizure will end within a few minutes and the person will enter a postseizure state of drowsiness, loss of memory, headache, confusion, etc. Excessive stimulation may aggravate the confused state; you should provide a quiet atmosphere for the person to "sleep it off" while keeping him propped up on one side so that any saliva can drain from the mouth. If (as only rarely happens) the seizure activity does not stop within three to four minutes, you should call for emergency transportation to the nearest medical facility.

Significance of Seizures

A given seizure can vary enormously in significance depending on age, other medical problems, and so on.

Seizures during high fevers are not unusual in children; once having occurred, the doctor will usually place the child on medication to be taken regularly or when a high temperature occurs. A seizure occurring for the first time in an adult (past age twenty-five) is more likely to signify some brain disease and should be investigated thoroughly by a good primary care physician and/or neurologist. Seizures that signify the disease called epilepsy can usually, but not always, be identified with brain wave studies (EEG's—electroencephalograms). The point is this: There are many different causes of seizures and the appropriate treatment will depend on the underlying cause. Any seizure occurring for the first time must be investigated.

Discrimination

Unfortunately, our society still discriminates all too often against people with epilepsy—one of causes of recurrent seizures. The vast majority of people with epilepsy can be rendered almost completely seizure-free with medication. Such people can function normally and must be restricted only from activity that might pose danger should they have another seizure—such as climbing to high places, swimming alone, and so forth. I would like to impress strongly on employers and schools that people with epilepsy can usually lead almost completely normal lives; they need not be singled out for special treatment if their drug treatment program is successful.

Rarely, recurrent seizures are difficult to control with drugs, and other treatment approaches (including brain surgery) must be considered. In such relatively rare instances, referral to a good medical center is worthwhile for complete evaluation and treatment decision.

Sickle-Cell Abnormalities

One of the "anemias" that deserves special mention is sickle-cell anemia. This anemia is more accurately described as a "hemoglobinopathy"—a disease affecting hemoglobin, the stuff in red blood cells that carries oxygen. There are many such diseases, affecting many different people. Sickle-cell disease, however, is one of the most important of these disorders since it afflicts a significant number of Black people with serious disability and suffering. I will discuss this disorder under the following headings.

Cause

All of the hemoglobinopathies are marked by abnormalities in the composition of the chains of amino acids that make up hemoglobin. The sequence of amino acids is under the control of genes; thus, a hemoglobinopathy is properly described as a hereditary (or genetic) disease since it results from abnormal genes from the parents. In the case of sickle-cell disease, a change in only *one* of the 146 amino acids of one of the chains in the hemoglobin molecule (and there are 200–300 million hemoglobin molecules in *each* red blood cell) causes all the trouble. This single change causes the red blood cell to assume a sickle (crescent) shape under certain conditions (such as low oxygen supply) and such abnormally shaped red cells are more easily destroyed than normal cells causing the "anemia" part of the disease. More significant, such cells plug up the circulation in smaller blood vessels causing the many manifestations of the disease described as sickle-cell "crises"—joint pains which may mimic arthritis, abdominal pains and shock which may mimic a serious surgical problem, plugging of the blood supply to the heart or brain which might imitate heart attacks and strokes, etc. It is obvious from this last sentence that sickle-cell disease is a very serious medical problem.

At this point it is absolutely critical to understand the difference between sickle-cell *disease* and sickle-cell *trait*. The disease is a condition in which abnormal genes have been inherited from *both* parents; the technical term for this pattern of inheritance (both parents) is *homozygous* inheritance. It is this kind of inheritance which causes the disease, the serious problem described above; such disease affects less than one percent of the Black population of this country.

In sickle-cell *trait,* only *one* abnormal gene (from one of the parents) has been inherited; such an inheritance pattern is called *heterozygous.* Inheriting only one abnormal gene makes all the difference in the world. Such persons have much less abnormal hemoglobin in their red blood cells and therefore are much less likely to form sickle-shaped cells; only under extreme conditions of low oxygen will such cells be found. People with the trait (versus the disease) are described as carriers—i.e., they have an abnormal gene but they will not know it without appropriate testing since they usually have no symptoms. The trait is much more common, affecting about nine percent of Blacks in this country.

Screening

I have taken this much time to discuss basic genetics because there is considerable controversy in our country about screening tests for Black people. Screening tests are tests which can detect a carrier; in the case of sickle-cell trait, a simple blood test can demonstrate the presence of an abnormal gene in somebody who would not otherwise know it. The significance of such information is that, if *one* parent is a carrier, there is no chance that any of their children will get the *disease*, though some of them may also become carriers—may have the trait. However, if *both* parents are carriers, even though they themselves are healthy, there is a one in four chance in any pregnancy that their children will get the disease—the serious form which produces all the problems described above and which usually results in death at an early age. Thus, many Black people anticipating parenthood would like to know what the chances are that their children will get sickle-cell disease or trait. Given such information, they may wish to make a decision not to have their own children but instead to consider adoption.

The controversy surrounding screening lies in a discussion of whether such screening should be mandatory and whether resulting information will be more troublesome than it is worth. For example, if screening is done on Black children and they are found to have the trait (which, after all, will not hurt them—only possibly any children they might have), will such information label them as being "abnormal" in a way which might harm their development? Another example would be an adult who is denied a job or insurance because of the label "sickle cell" in his record. I won't pretend to answer these important questions, but I will say that, in my own experience, Blacks who understand the problems as I have outlined them and who are anticipating parenthood are often eager to gain such information.

Diagnosis and Treatment of the Disease

Sickle-cell *disease* will usually manifest itself early in life as "crises" begin to develop. Occasionally, a person with the disease will not have symptoms until adulthood—but that is rare. Diagnosis depends on suspecting sickle-cell disease in any Black with symptoms of the kind described above (plus many other possible symptoms). The final diagnosis is made by specific blood tests.

Unfortunately, there is no cure for the disease. Many things can be done to help alleviate the symptoms—blood transfusions, pain medications, oxygen, etc. Urea has been tried in treatment of acute crises, but there is no good evidence that it is better than other forms of treatment. As mentioned earlier, most people with the disease die in early adulthood.

This grim description reinforces the significance of screening and the possibility of family planning. Further information on sickle-cell disease can be obtained from the National Association for Sickle-Cell Disease, 945 South Western Avenue, Suite 206, Los Angeles, California 90006.

Sinus Infections

Two things are important to say about sinus infections. First, it is important to make a definite diagnosis. And, second, it is crucial to seek expert therapy. Thousands of people suffer unnecessarily because of improper diagnosis and/or treatment. Now comes the bad news: it is often difficult to diagnose and effectively treat sinusitis—especially chronic "low-grade" infections.

Diagnosis involves *careful* examination of the nose and throat—not just a casual look-in. Sometimes a primary care physician will do a thorough job, but usually a visit to an ENT specialist is required; unfortunately, their charges are often high but if the symptoms are troublesome and persistent the money may be well spent. Somewhere in the diagnostic process, sinus X rays must be taken.

Treatment depends on whether the infection is in an acute (many symptoms, fever, pain, high white blood count, etc.) or chronic (no fever, minimal but annoying symptoms) stage. Acute treatment involves antibiotics, pain and decongestant medications, and other supportive measures. If appropriate antibiotics are chosen—and cultures often are not helpful—acute infections will usually get better quickly.

I wish I could say the same about treatment of chronic infection. It is in this situation that conservative surgical procedures to promote drainage are often useful. (Surgery or any manipulation of sinuses during acute infections is a no-no.)

The basic problem with sinusitis is that it is often confused with other conditions that may easily overlap—generalized colds, tooth infections, allergic conditions of the nose, etc. That is why careful diagnosis is required. And that is why the ENT specialist is often worth his fee (at least in this instance). However, be suspicious of any high-priced treatment requiring you to come back to the office every week for a quick check or "painting" or application of some magic liquid. A good specialist should be more decisive and clearly able to help or not.

Skin Problems

There are three basic questions to be answered when you develop a skin problem:

1. Is the problem confined to the skin—or is it symptomatic of underlying disease?

2. Is it an infectious or contagious problem requiring antibiotics?

3. Would this skin problem benefit from the special skills of a dermatologist?

Let's start with the last question first. You might well ask: Why not automatically go to a dermatologist (specialist in skin diseases) when the problem seems to be the skin? The answer: A dermatologist is often expensive and sometimes not necessary. Most skin problems can be handled by primary care physicians—internists, pediatricians, family physicians—at considerably less expense. Indeed, some physicians joke that all one needs to be a dermatologist is a big vat of "triple cream"—a name for the many medicinal creams on the market (requiring a prescription) which contain three different kinds of drugs, making the cream a kind of shotgun therapy which will cure almost anything. Certainly that's an exaggeration— but I think it's a safe rule to suggest that all skin problems should be seen first by a primary care physician.

Having said this, let me rescue myself from proper criticism by pointing out that many primary care physicians are ill-equipped to handle more than the most common and routine skin problems. (Skin disease is one of the neglected areas in most medical schools and even post– medical school training programs in primary care disciplines are commonly deficient in dermatology.) Given the great importance of the skin to both physical appearance and consequent psychological well being, it must be emphasized that there are many skin problems which *should* be seen by a well-trained and up-to-date dermatologist. (I emphasize such a description because dermatology is one of those specialties that can be practiced entirely outside the hospital and be, therefore, free from hospital controls and standards. Some older practitioners who call themselves dermatologists have not had thorough training. You need to check on credentials.) Specifically, the following merit the attention of a dermatologist:

1. *Severe Acne:* This common skin problem presents both a medical and psychological challenge to any physician. While the cause is still not absolutely clear, great strides have been made in treatment. Long-term treatment with broad-spectrum antibiotics (such as tetracycline) remains one of the cornerstones of therapy, but other therapies can be used—and a dermatologist's help can be crucial in difficult cases.

2. *Severe Psoriasis:* Again, cause and treatment of this common and often disabling disease are more elusive than we would like, but treatment methods are changing and a specialist is in order for at least periodic consultation. Recently, Harvard dermatologists announced a dramatic breakthrough in treatment involving the oral taking of a drug followed by exposure to newly developed longwave ultraviolet light sources. The "breakthrough" involved, apart from excellent results, is the use of an oral medication (versus smearing coal-tar over the body) thus leading to the possibility of a simple, office type of treatment. It must be emphasized that this treatment is still experimental and not yet available to the public.

3. *Any persistent skin problem:* Since very few skin problems are life-threatening, most can stand the "test of time." But when a problem becomes persistently annoying and has not responded to the therapy offered by a primary physician, a trip to a carefully selected dermatologist may well be worth the money spent. The key is to find one who is well-trained; usually your primary health care source can advise you.

The first two questions posed at the beginning of this section are questions that any physician who sees you with a skin problem must attempt to answer. Some skin problems are manifestations of serious underlying disease; a good primary care physician should be alert to these possibilities. Many skin problems represent infectious bacterial disease requiring antibiotics; again, a good primary care physician should handle this without problem. However, most skin problems turn out to be eczematous dermatitis —a delayed hypersensitivity reaction to external or internal inciting agents: sprays, food, poison ivy, soaps, cosmetics, etc. The list is endless; sometimes the offending substance is obvious, but more often the culprit is difficult to pinpoint. Fortunately, most are responsive to symptomatic treatment coupled with avoidance of the offending agent(s).

Finally, a word of tribute to our skin—a remarkable covering and protecting device, one that is continually abused by overexposure to external environment. Common sense should tell us to avoid extremes, whether it be sun or soap. But, where appearance is involved, the human animal seems to operate according to anything but common sense.

The following are brief discussions of some of the more common skin problems encountered by all of us.

Boils and Carbuncles

These terms are used interchangeably by lay people even though they do have a technical difference. A boil (also called a furuncle) represents an infection of a hair follicle and surrounding tissue; when several boils collect together the resulting mess is called a carbuncle. Whatever you call these collections of pus, they are troublesome at best and potentially dangerous. Localized infections which occur in the so-called dangerous triangle formed by the corners of the upper lip and the nose should not be pinched or squeezed since such manipulation may (though rarely lead to serious brain infections.

A small pimple or two can usually be managed without paying for medical attention; time will usually take care of the problem—and hotpacking may speed up the process of "coming to a head" and draining spontaneously. If boils are widespread, even though small, antibiotics are usually required to bring the situation under control.

And, when a localized situation reaches the larger stage of a carbuncle, an "I&D" (incision and drainage) is usually required. I have seen many people suffer unnecessarily with a large, painful, oozing carbuncle, hoping that it will go away; most will never clear up until an opening is made allowing adequate draining. Unless the carbuncle is very large or located in a critical place, this can usually be accomplished painlessly under local anesthesia; rarely, such carbuncles have to be opened and drained in the operating room.

A surgeon or primary care physician who does minor surgery is the person to see. If such help cannot be obtained readily, a trip to an emergency facility is justified since these situations represent real discomfort and potential danger.

Skin Tumors

Skin cancer is the most common cancer of the human race; it is, also, one of the most curable—*if* detected early. Which is to say that it is a cancer for which we as individuals bear great responsibility. That responsibility begins with proper care of the skin, particularly in relation to sunlight. There is no question that excessive, long-term exposure to sun increases the incidence of skin cancer, especially in light-skinned individuals who burn easily and tan with difficulty.

Most troublesome are the "moles" that all of us have. When should we be concerned? Honesty compels me to say that there is no absolutely certain way to say in a given instance whether cancer is involved short of biopsy —looking at the tissue under a microscope. Fortunately, an experienced physician can usually judge as to which skin lesions (abnormalities) need to be biopsied. In the meantime, the primary responsibility lies with the individual to identify any skin mark or growth that is new, changing (growing, bleeding, changing color, etc.), or just "looks bad." Take no chances—that's the "rule." If a skin lesion looks suspicious, a surgeon (general or plastic) or dermatologist is the best physician with whom to check.

Rashes

Skin rashes are part of life—rare is the person who has never had one (or more). And their causes are as varied as life itself—infection, allergy, irritants. Sometimes, the cause cannot be determined and the rash must be treated symptomatically.

Generally rashes can be divided into two categories of concern—those accompanied by other symptoms of illness such as fever, swollen glands, and general ill-feeling, and those confined to the local annoyance (itching, etc.) of the rash itself. The former must be considered as part of the total disease process and treated as such; the latter can usually be managed more casually with a good home-try at relieving the discomfort with prescribed creams, antihistamines, etc.

Persistent or recurrent rashes merit more intensive investigation for serious underlying disease. Usually a primary care physician (internist or pediatrician, depending on age—or family physician) is the place to begin. It may be necessary to consult a dermatologist and/or allergist; but look for guidance from your primary care physician.

Itching (*Pruritus*)

Itching is the most common reason for people seeking the help of a dermatologist. While itching is usually not life-threatening (though in rare cases it may be a signal of serious disease) it can be devastatingly annoying—one of those burdens of life that can "drive you up a wall."

Apart from reaction to stress (so-called psychogenic causes), most generalized itching is due to an allergic reaction to one of many things—direct irritants, sunlight, food, drugs, etc. If the itching is very mild and not associated with other problems, it may be handled in the short run with home remedies—hot or cool compresses, tub soaking, etc. Over-the-counter remedies should generally be avoided since they often make the problem worse, but time-tested home creams may help. If the itching is severe or extensive, a search for more serious, underlying medical problems is in order.

Smoking

While I have referred to smoking many times elsewhere in this book, I think it would be useful to draw it all together at one point—as follows:

The major medical reasons to stop cigarette smoking include:

1. A twenty to twenty-five times greater chance of lung cancer, which kills ninety-five percent of its victims in the first five years.

2. A two to three times greater chance of dying from a heart attack, the nation's number one killer.

3. A greater chance of developing chronic lung disease —emphysema—the most common and debilitating chronic disease of the human race.

4. A greater chance of developing poor circulation to the extremities.

5. A greater chance of burning to death.

6. A greater chance that your children will smoke.

Not to mention the cost and the smell.

So what should someone do who wants to quit smoking?

I don't have any better answers than anyone else. But I will offer the following inputs to your possible interest in the subject.

1. One famous thoracic surgeon (who has made a good living because people smoke) suggests that we miss part of the danger of smoking because we don't use the organ of our bodies best able to detect toxic fumes. He suggests that people smoke through their nose instead of their mouth. He claims such an approach has caused several people to quit. You may wish to try it.

2. Some people use the excuse that the damage has already been done and it won't pay to quit. That may be true if a lung cancer has already started to grow. But if not, it definitely pays to quit. Within weeks, lung function tests start to improve, taste improves, and the usual chronic cough decreases or disappears. Ask someone who has quit if you don't believe me.

3. Some people say that if they quit they will gain weight and that's just as bad for your health. Wrong. You may gain weight initially, but any weight gain (even a hundred pounds) is a better health risk by far than smoking. My advice is to tackle one problem at a time: Quit smoking and then tackle any weight gain that might result. The problem is that we can see those extra pounds but we can't see the growing lung cancer until it is too late.

4. Some people say that, since they have to die anyway, they might as well die from smoking. Two problems with that argument: While we all expect to die, we usually don't want premature death, which smoking certainly promotes; and dying from lung cancer is one of the worst ways to go.

I have been increasingly impressed with hypnosis as a method of both weight and smoking control. You might give it consideration if you have access to a competent hypnotist whose fee you can afford.

We are all aware of the statistics which indicate that more people are smoking than ever—a "tribute" to the advertising and tobacco industries of this country. But millions of people (including a large number of physicians) have quit. Why not you?

Sore Throat

There is nothing quite so annoying as a sore throat—for both patient and doctor. While most sore throats are not serious and will get better with time, they make us feel miserable far beyond their medical significance; every time we swallow it feels as though a gremlin is rubbing the back of our throats with sandpaper.

The doctor is disturbed by sore throats because—while he knows that the vast majority are caused by a virus and therefore will get better *without* being treated with antibiotics—he really can't be sure that a streptococcal bacteria (strep throat) is not the cause without doing a throat culture. And making sure that a sore throat is not due to strep is what it's all about. The problem with a strep throat is not the sore throat itself but the damage the strep germ may do to the heart or kidneys if it is not eradicated by penicillin or other appropriate antibiotic. Most rheumatic heart disease and some chronic kidney disease could be prevented if strep throats were promptly treated.

So what's a mother (or anyone) to do about all the sore throats of life? *The only safe course is to culture any sore throat that persists beyond twenty-four hours.* I know I'm going to get arguments on that statement, but I'm only telling you what I would do for myself or members of my family. It's easy to take chances but a culture is so simple (and *usually* cheap) that it's penny-wise and pound-foolish not to get one. (Many communities provide free cultures to children under a certain age.)

Notice that I did not say that everyone with a sore throat should be treated with penicillin. There are those doctors who simply skip the culture and give everyone with a sore throat a course of penicillin. If there is any question as to follow-up, that approach may be justified, but a much better approach is as follows: (1) culture all sore throats lasting more than twenty-four hours regardless of appearance; (2) if the sore throat is accompanied by high fever and/or pus is seen in the tonsillar area, start a course of penicillin and await the culture results before deciding whether to continue the full course; (3) if the throat is simply red and there is no high fever, await the culture results before starting antibiotics.

One warning word to patients: Be sure to complete the

course of antibiotics as prescribed. (Normally penicillin is the antibiotic of choice, but there are others that can be used for the person allergic to penicillin.) Antibiotics for a strep throat should be taken for a minimum of ten days. Even though you should feel better in one or two days it is *very important* to complete the ten-day or two-week course to insure complete elimination of the strep bacteria.

If a sore throat is due to a virus, there's not much you can do except try to make it feel better with aspirin, gargle, lozenges, etc. With such measures you will probably feel better in about seven days; otherwise it will take about a week. (Sorry about that old gag.)

Strokes (CVA's)

First, some terminology is in order. Most lay people use the term "stroke" to refer to an episode in which a person rather suddenly changes in ability to move and/or talk; sometimes these changes are very dramatic but quite often they are subtle and may be noticed only by close friends and relatives. When the episode is very sudden and dramatic, the term "shock" ("my mother had a shock") is sometimes used.

Doctors use these two terms in a more specific application. "Strokes" refer to a wide range of neurological symptoms that result from impairment of circulation to the brain; another way to describe this is to call the event a "cerebrovascular accident"—the "CVA" you may have heard doctors talk about. "Shock" has a very different meaning to a doctor; the term refers to a generalized (all over the body) problem with circulation in which many vital tissues (including the brain) are not getting enough blood.

From now on, I will use the term "stroke" to mean a

problem in the blood vessels *leading to* and the vessels *in* the brain, causing problems with the normal circulation of blood to brain tissue and resulting in damage to that brain tissue which expresses that damage by many possible symptoms—damaged speech, inability to use various parts of the body, blindness, etc. (Please read that complicated sentence again because from now on I'm going to say "stroke" to mean all of that.)

Actually, there are many things that can go wrong in the vessels leading to or in the brain. But, for our purposes, I will list the three major ways in which circulation may be impaired.

1. *Thrombosis:* The word thrombosis means a "clot," so the phrase "cerebral thrombosis" refers to a clot in a vessel(s) of the brain. Actually, many clots that cause strokes occur in vessels leading *to* the brain (see the following discussion) rather than in vessels *in* the brain. It is easy to visualize how a clot would interrupt blood flow beyond the point of the clot and cause a stroke as we defined it above. The major cause of such clot formation is that same process that causes a coronary thrombosis (heart attack)—namely atherosclerosis. When we talk about the prevention of heart disease, then, what we say also applies to the prevention of strokes— since the underlying process is the same.

2. *Embolus:* An embolus is a "traveling clot." So a "cerebral embolus" is a stroke caused by a clot from somewhere downstream which travels in the vessels leading to the brain and gets caught somewhere blocking circulation beyond that point. One of the causes of such traveling clots is the formation of a thrombosis from which a piece of clot breaks off.

3. *Hemorrhage:* This refers to a situation in which a blood vessel actually breaks causing both direct destruction of brain tissue and obvious interruption of circulation. The most common cause of such breaking is the rupture of a vessel weakened by hypertension and atherosclerosis. Indeed, hypertension plays a more prominent role in this type of stroke than atherosclerosis. Sometimes, a blood vessel will rupture because of a weakness in a vessel that was probably present from birth; you may have heard this referred to as a "congenital aneurysm."

By now you should have gotten the idea that this "stroke" business is very complicated. In fact, a careful diagnosis of the cause and "location" (i.e., which vessels are involved) of stroke symptoms often requires great knowledge and skill; neurologists are the experts often called in on difficult stroke cases. There are controversies in the diagnosis and treatment of the various kinds of strokes; a discussion of these controversies is way beyond the scope of this book. When and if you are confronted with a stroke situation in your family, you are going to have to rely on the advice and explanation of a good primary care physician and the expert consultants (neurologists and neurosurgeons) that he may wish to call in.

There are, however, two areas that every person should know something about. I would like to direct your attention to these areas now.

Stroke Prevention (*Including Transient Ischemic Attacks*)
I have already alluded to two areas of stroke prevention —namely, reducing factors which promote atherosclerosis (so-called hardening of the arteries) and treating hypertension. (You should read the section on "risk factors" in

the section on coronary artery disease; what is said there about preventing atherosclerosis applies here also.)

I would, however, like to comment on a phenomenon which applies specifically to stroke prevention—namely transient ischemic attacks (usually referred to as TIA's). A "TIA" refers to an episode (attack) which is transient (gets better usually within ten minutes though it can be shorter or longer) and is presumed to be caused by temporarily decreased circulation (ischemia) to the brain. In other words, a TIA is a kind of "ministroke" or "temporary stroke" which reverses itself. The importance of TIA's is that they *may* herald the coming of a stroke which *might* be prevented with medical and/or surgical therapy.

Obviously this subject is complex; you can tell by the way I am emphasizing the qualifying words. The most basic statement I can make is this; If you experience *any* kind of temporary loss or change in function—blindness, change in speech, confusion, difficulty in doing calculations, dizziness, etc.—you should check it out with your primary care physician. This becomes even more necessary as you get older. Most of the time, an impending stroke will *not* be the cause. But this is a determination for your doctor to make—not you.

The reason I stress all this is that in a significant number of cases where examination and tests demonstrate that circulation to the brain is indeed the cause of these temporary attacks, preventative therapy may be very helpful. Specifically, two forms of therapy are used—anticoagulant drugs and surgery to either remove or bypass the clot causing the symptoms. Surgery is used only for problems in vessels accessible to and suitable for surgical repair; this almost always means vessels in the neck rather than vessels in the brain. The tests required to make these decisions are sometimes difficult and potentially dangerous

—particularly angiography, which involves the injection of dye into the vessels leading to the brain. You must rely on the skill and judgment of your physicians; at the point where surgery becomes a possibility and angiography is therefore required, a neurologist and/or neurosurgeon should be a part of the picture. (Sometimes a general vascular surgeon does surgery on the vessels of the neck which lead to the brain.) All I can really describe here is the situation of temporary symptoms which mean you *must* see a doctor; don't take chances.

A quick word of warning. Anticoagulant drugs (blood-thinners) and/or surgery on vessels leading to the brain should never be offered casually without careful examination and appropriate studies. At the very least, a neurological exam (checking sensation and movement all over the body), checking the vessels in the neck (feeling and listening with a stethoscope), looking in the back of the eyes and testing the blood pressure in the vessels of the eye (ophthalmodynamometry is the name of this test)—these should all be a part of the examination. Surgery should never be done without angiography (X rays taken with dye injected into the vessels in question) being done first. It is unlikely that you will encounter physicians who will recommend anticoagulant drugs and/or surgery without careful examination. But if someone seems in a big rush—be suspicious. Your best guide is a good primary care physician you have reason to trust.

Stroke Treatment

Once a stroke has occurred and the patient survives the initial crisis, the question becomes: What, if any, will be the progress over the next weeks, months, even years? There are no simple answers to that all-important question. There are some general guidelines that all physicians have in mind but I will not even mention them here because there are so many individual variations. What can and should be said here is that the help of good rehabilitation facilities may make the difference between mere survival and a reasonable life-style. The Task Force on Strokes initiated by the National Institutes of Health is promoting the concept of a "stroke team"—a multidisciplinary approach to the rehabilitation of the stroke victim. Many medical institutions today have such facilities under the direction of a physiatrist—a doctor who specializes in rehabilitation. If a member of your family suffers a stroke and survives, ask about rehabilitation possibilities. If the answers are vague or absent, check with your local or state health department for advice. The matter is worth pursuing.

Thrombophlebitis

First, a little terminology is in order. *Phlebitis* means "inflammation of a vein." *Thrombus* means "a blood clot." The two terms together obviously refer to a blood clot inside a vein with associated inflammation of that vein. This process can occur in any of the veins in our body, but the most common location is the veins of the lower leg, and it is this entity (leg vein thrombophlebitis) that I will be discussing in this section.

Before proceeding to a systematic discussion of this important topic, I wish to make clear the distinction between thrombophlebitis and a bruise. (I am spending time on this distinction because the considerable publicity given to thrombophlebitis has understandably raised anxiety levels about all "blood clots" of the leg.) By definition, a bruise is also a "blood clot" of sorts—i.e. an abnormal collection of blood in a place where it shouldn't be. However, a bruise represents a blood clot *outside* a blood vessel; it is therefore not dangerous in the sense of producing a clot which can "travel" in the blood vessel system to other parts of the body. A bruise represents a collection of blood which has escaped from damaged blood vessels (usually very small ones) into the surrounding tissue outside the vessels. A bruise may be painful and look awful— and in rare instances it may be dangerous because of secondary infection or actual blood loss (in a very large hematoma). But most bruises disappear with time, though the color changes over a period of weeks may rival the fall foliage. Again, they do not present the danger of a traveling clot (embolus) so feared with blood clots *inside* vessels.

Finally, we must make the important distinction between thrombophlebitis of the surface (superficial) and deep veins of the legs. The problem can arise in either of these two venous systems. When it occurs in the superficial veins, symptoms are usually obvious—tenderness and redness along the course of the vein. Superficial thrombophlebitis, while often painful and frightening, is seldom dangerous, because large clots are unlikely to break off and travel to the lungs. It is, however, important to treat such superficial disease (local heat and bed rest with the leg elevated) to prevent the process from extending up the leg to the junction with the deep veins at the very upper part of the leg; if the clot-inflammation process extends to that junction, it may extend into the deep veins where the possibility of large clots breaking off and traveling is much greater.

Now that we've got our focus narrowed to thrombophlebitis of the deep veins, we can discuss it under the following important headings:

Cause and Prevention

Right at the start I must say that we don't know exactly what causes T-P (as I will hereafter refer to deep-vein thrombophlebitis). We do know, however, that it is associated with several conditions which involve a "stasis" (stagnation, slowing) of blood flow in the veins of the leg: pregnancy (increased pressure on the veins of the pelvis reduces return flow from the legs); confinement to bed (particularly dangerous postoperatively); prolonged sitting or standing (the muscles of the legs are not moving and pushing blood in the veins back toward the heart), among others. The obvious prevention for these conditions is to prevent stasis—get the patient to move the legs as soon as possible after an operation, wear elastic stockings to prevent pooling of blood in the leg veins, etc.

Birth control pills have been associated with an increased incidence of T-P. In order to put this in proper perspective, it should be emphasized that the state of pregnancy (which the pill very effectively prevents) has an even higher risk of T-P than the use of the pill. But the pill should not be taken by anyone who has ever had or who develops T-P; another form of contraception should be used. (Be sure to change methods of contraception under the guidance of a knowledgeable source so that pregnancy does not occur in the changeover period.)

Anyone who has had T-P once is at higher risk to develop it again—though most do not. Such a person should be especially careful to avoid conditions associated with the development of T-P. Factors in addition to those mentioned include obesity, anemia, shock, dehydration, and infection.

Symptoms—Diagnosis

The problem is that about half of the people with proven T-P have no symptoms. (In fact, it is conjectured that most of us have episodes of very minor T-P at some time in our life without ever knowing it.) Sometimes T-P is not diagnosed until it shows itself by its major complication—an embolus (traveling blood clot).

Many people do have symptoms—ranging from a vague feeling of heaviness in the leg to obvious pain and swelling in the leg. This is one of those conditions in medicine that require a strong degree of suspicion on the part of the patient.

In most cases, diagnosis can be made on the basis of a good physical exam by a knowledgeable primary care physician. By "good" I mean careful searching for pain and tenderness, movement of the leg and foot to elicit pain, and measuring of the legs for swelling that may not be obvious to the naked eye.

In some cases, the diagnosis of T-P will not be certain even after careful exam. The expert then has several diagnostic aids to fall back on—scans, impedance studies, ultrasound (all noninvasive—that is, not involving puncture of the skin) and venograms (sometimes called phlebograms), which involve injecting dye into the veins of the leg and taking X rays to outline the veins. Rarely, even after the use of these techniques, a diagnosis may not be absolutely certain, but treatment will be started since the risks of treatment are generally less than the risk of possible traveling clots.

Treatment

The object of treatment is to prevent the breaking loose of a clot which might travel to the lungs (after passing through the right side of the heart) and interfere with circulation of blood through the lungs. (See following discussion of pulmonary embolus.) There are four major ways in which this is achieved:

Local measures: As soon as the diagnosis of T-P has been made, *complete* bed rest with leg elevation is *mandatory*. It is not mere rhetoric to call acute thrombophlebitis a medical emergency. Aside from the use of intravenous medication as described below, hospitalization is necessary to assure bed rest. The rationale for such rest is to allow time for the clot to adhere to the inflamed wall of the vein, thereby reducing the chance that it might break away; any movement interferes with this process. After five to ten days of successful treatment, walking (not standing or sitting) can be slowly started.

Anticoagulant drugs: There are two major kinds of drugs which prevent clot formation: heparin, which cannot be taken orally, and various oral agents suitable for long-term use. In the acute phase, heparin (which is given by needle either intravenously or subcutaneously) is definitely the best drug to prevent the possibility of a pulmonary embolus (blood clot to the lung). The questions of how long to continue heparin, when and if to start oral drugs, how long to take oral drugs—these must be considered individually for any given patient and course of events. A skillful primary care physician is required. There is also renewed interest in the use of aspirin (salicylates) for long-term anticoagulation.

Thrombolytic drugs: These drugs act to "dissolve" clots (versus prevent formation of clots). There has been a great deal of interest in this kind of drug in recent years and studies generally have indicated their usefulness. They are still not widely used but will probably become a standard part of therapy in the next few years.

Surgical intervention: Various techniques to block the passage of clots from the legs to the lungs can be used in patients who cannot take the drugs described above (for example, very recent surgical patients who might bleed easily or patients with active ulcers that might bleed) or who are not responding to drug therapy. Such surgery is not without hazard, but, in the face of recurrent emboli, the risk of surgery is often less than the risk of a fatal blood clot. Rarely, a massive blood clot which has not responded to other forms of therapy will be directly removed from the vein.

Pulmonary Embolus (Blood Clot to Lung)

The most common cause of this serious medical problem is thrombophlebitis of the legs. Such clots (hereafter referred to as PE) cause problems by blocking the flow of blood through the lungs; if the clots are large enough to block a significant amount of blood flow the result is similar to suffocation in the sense that the body cannot get enough oxygen to its tissues. (Indeed, in severe cases of PE the symptoms are often similar to suffocation—the person turns blue and gasps for breath.) The so-called massive PE is a frightening emergency (the blue, gasping patient), and the death rate is very high. Heroic measures are required to save a life—including quick and dramatic surgical intervention to remove the clot.

More common and more difficult to diagnose are smaller clots which cause less obvious symptoms. Difficulty breathing, coughing with or without blood, pain during breathing, unexplained anxiety about breathing—these are possible ways in which a lung blood clot may present its symptoms. Most often, tests will be required to make the diagnosis. Blood drawn from an artery (instead of the usual vein) for determination of oxygen content is often used as a kind of screening test. But various X ray and scan studies—including studies in which dye is injected directly into the lung blood vessels—are usually necessary to make the diagnosis.

Treatment involves anticoagulant drugs and other emergency measures as required—oxygen, drugs for shock, surgery, etc. Long-term anticoagulant therapy may be necessary.

Chronic Venous Insufficiency

Since this condition is most commonly a sequel to phlebitis, it is appropriate to briefly mention it in this section. The major point to be made is that the best treatment is prevention—which means vigorous treatment of acute phlebitis and the use of leg elevation and elastic stockings whenever possible during and after acute phlebitis.

The process of phlebitis often destroys the valves of leg veins; this prevents emptying of leg veins during walking and exercise, as would normally occur. The resulting increased venous pressure leads to the common secondary changes in the skin (thinning, color changes, shiny texture)—which eventually lead to ulceration. Once this stage is reached, treatment becomes much more difficult and reversal is seldom achieved; brownish color changes of the skin never go away.

So, again, the message is preventative care. People with such venous difficulties should take advantage of every opportunity to elevate their legs and to wear elastic and/or support stockings. These simple measures have great effectiveness.

Tonsillectomy and Adenoidectomy (T&A)

I assume everyone has gotten the message that "T&A's" are no longer being done just because the tonsils and adenoids are there. But there is still evidence of unnecessary T&A's, so the message is worth repeating: The indications for such surgery are much more restrictive than twenty years ago, and the operation is now considered more of a last than a first resort.

Let's be honest. Many T&A's were done in the past for quick financial gain. However, honesty also requires the statement that many physicians genuinely believed that the tonsils were relatively useless appendages in the throat and should be gotten rid of at the first sign of trouble.

Unfortunately, the evidence concerning the role and usefulness of the tonsils is still not clear. There are suggestions (but *not* clearly proven) that the tonsils do play a useful role in the defense system of the body. What is clear, however, is that tonsilar infection can be adequately controlled in most cases by antibiotics (see Sore Throat) thus avoiding the cost and risk of surgery.

Having said this, it must be said that there are some very legitimate reasons to take out the tonsils and/or the adenoids. (It is important that these two different tissues be considered separately both in terms of diagnosis and any necessary surgery; they should not be automatically taken out together.) Included in such reasons are:

1. Prior abscesses, which almost always will recur otherwise

2. Airway obstruction sufficient to cause breathing problems for the child

3. Any suspicion of malignancy

4. Certain cases of persistent fluid in the ears (the adenoids are usually the problem)

5. Recurrent infections of such severity and frequency as to cause unreasonable loss of school or work time.

In other words, each situation must be treated individually. When either a tonsillectomy or adenoidectomy or both are proposed, ask the big question: Why?

Thyroid Disease

The thyroid gland sits in the front part of the neck. Like many other glands in our body, it has wide-ranging effects on the metabolism of our bodies. The complexities of thyroid disease are the subject of entire textbooks; for this book, the following summary information is most important.

Many ills of mankind are blamed on "my thyroid." Most commonly, excess weight is attributed to "my glands" or "my thyroid." The signs of deranged metabolism, however, are usually more than such things as fatigue or excess weight—and today much of the guesswork concerning our metabolism has been eliminated by the use of sophisticated tests which can measure thyroid function very accurately. The day of gross BMR (basal metabolism rate) measurements is gone.

Basically, diseases of the thyroid cause either overactive (hyperthyroid) or underactive (hypothyroid) metabolic responses. Classically, the hyperthyroid individual manifests with sweating, weight loss, heat intolerance, nervousness, rapid heart rate, increased reflexes, bulging eyes, etc. In contrast, the hypothyroid individual presents with intolerance to cold, constipation, hoarseness, puffy skin, slow heart rate, sluggish reflexes, etc. However, many people with changed thyroid function may not have such obvious symptoms; thyroid hyper- or hypo-function may masquerade as other disease. For example, it is not uncommon for people to be labeled with psychiatric depression when they are in fact hypothyroid.

One of the common problems in medicine is that individual who was told years ago that he had "low thyroid" and was put on "thyroid pills." Many people so labeled and treated were not accurately diagnosed (tests available today were not around then) and have been taking unnecessary medicine without being rechecked. Anyone reading this who has been taking thyroid pills for years without being checked by a good primary care physician should make an appointment for such a check even as he or she reads this.

The opposite problem is represented by people who had their thyroids removed surgically years ago and have not had followup studies to make sure they have not become hypothyroid. Anyone who had thyroid surgery and has not had a check in years should do so. The same problem can arise from someone who had hyperthyroidism treated with radioactive iodine to destroy thyroid tissue; like surgical removal, such treatment can produce too much reduction in thyroid function.

Some thyroid diseases will produce visible and palpable changes in the thyroid gland which can be seen and felt during careful examination. Any physical examination should include a feel of the anterior neck. Cancer of the thyroid gland often presents with a painless lump or nodule; any swelling or lump in the anterior neck (besides the normal adam's apple) should be investigated. The diffuse enlargement of the gland (goiter) so common in days before iodized salt may still occasionally occur with certain forms of thyroid disease.

In summary, thyroid disease is a complex subject requiring special knowledge to diagnose and treat. Advances in diagnosis and treatment (new drugs, etc.) have been considerable. Anyone treated for thyroid disease many years ago but not recently should recheck with an appropriate physician.

Urinary Tract Problems

I am lumping several diseases together under this heading for this reason: Most people understand the urinary tract best in terms of its final product—namely, urine. In other words, if urination seems normal, all's well with the world—and vice versa. Which isn't too far from the medical summary of the situation.

Certain tests, besides the all-important urinalysis, are common in investigating problems of the urinary tract. They are worth mentioning:

1. *I.V.P.—Intravenous pyelogram:* This involves injecting dye into an arm vein and then taking abdominal X rays at intervals (usually during the next one to two hours). The dye is followed as it is concentrated in the kidneys and then excreted down the ureters (one from each kidney), collected in the bladder, and passed out through the single urethra to the "outside world." Thus this single exam provides valuable information both as to the function of the kidney and the anatomy of the entire urinary system—kidneys, ureters, bladder, and urethra. The test involves a minimal risk of allergic reaction; anyone with a suggestive allergic history (such as shellfish allergy) must be observed carefully during the procedure and even pretested.

2. *Retrograde pyelogram:* This involves inserting small tubes (catheters) up into the ureters to the kidney and

then injecting dye to outline the urinary system; since the dye comes from "below" instead of through the normal pathway of urine formation, the procedure is called a retrograde ("backward") pyelogram. In the male, the insertion of the catheters via the penis causes enough discomfort to usually warrant doing the procedure under light anesthesia in the hospital; in the female, local anesthesia with xylocaine jelly is often sufficient. Though much less common than the IVP, this procedure is done for many legitimate reasons including the necessity of visualizing the urinary system in people who for various reasons (including allergy to dye injected intravenously) cannot have an IVP.

3. *Cystoscopy:* This involves gently inserting a tube into the bladder via the urethra, which is very short in the female and longer via the penis in the male. It can often be done as an office procedure. It provides both a look at the bladder (giving much information not obtainable by X-ray studies) and a way of removing tissue (or tumors) from the bladder.

There are two kinds of doctors who take care of urinary tract problems. Most primary care physicians—including gynecologists—handle nonsurgical problems of the urinary system. A nephrologist is a subspecialist of internal medicine who handles more difficult nonsurgical problems—such as kidney failure. The urologist is a surgical subspecialist who treats many medical problems (like urinary tract infections) but is qualified to perform surgical procedures of the urinary system. Obviously there is considerable overlap as to who does what and the direction of a good primary physician is essential in complicated problems of the urinary tract.

Having given this general information I would now like

to list some of the more common diseases affecting the urinary tract and zero in on essential information for each.

Glomerulonephritis

This large word refers to a complicated process that affects both kidneys and is most commonly a sequel to a strep infection of the throat or skin; many other causes of this process are now known but antecedent strep infection is still the most important. And once glomerulonephritis occurs no specific treatment is possible, though it is still desirable to eradicate any strep germ in the body with penicillin or other appropriate antibiotics.

The real message of this disease is prevention. And prevention means eradicating any strep infections *before* the kidneys become involved. As explained in the section on sore throats, the reason for aggressively treating strep throats is not so much the damage to the throat but the prevention of subsequent damage by the strep germ to the heart (rheumatic fever) and kidneys (glomerulonephritis). About ten to fifteen percent of children and young adults with strep infections will develop kidney problems. In children under six, impetigo—skin infection—is the most common antecedent strep infection; in children over six (and adults) the typical strep throat is the most common antecedent. So, again, either of these manifestations of strep infection must be treated with antibiotics promptly— to protect the heart and kidneys.

If kidney disease does occur, it may manifest with symptoms—headache, malaise, puffiness of the eyes and face, bloody urine, etc. In many cases, however, symptoms are so mild that the disease is never suspected; only a urinalysis showing red cells, casts, and protein would make the diagnosis. Only a small percent of cases of glomerulonephritis go on to kidney failure—which leads to the terrible problems of dialysis and renal transplants. But most physicians feel that many of these tragic cases could be prevented if strep infections were treated early enough.

Such kidney failure is not to be confused with acute (sudden) kidney failure due to many possible causes—poisons (carbon tetrachloride, etc.), trauma (severe accidents), poor circulation (which causes a special form of kidney failure), etc. These acute forms are often more successful in outcome if the acute episode can be managed properly; the skills of specialists and critical care nursing are essential in these situations and transfer to such a medical center is mandatory.

Urinary Tract Infections (U.T.I.)

Infections of the urinary tract (hereinafter referred to as U.T.I.) are so common and potentially so serious that it is important you understand the basics of the subject.

Acute U.T.I.'s usually cause symptoms severe enough to promote a visit to the doctor; the most common symptom is frequent and painful urination, but other symptoms—fever, back or abdominal pain, nausea, and vomiting (particularly in children and females), may be prominent. The key elements in successful treatment of such acute episodes are the following:

1. *Accurate identification of the bacteria involved:* This involves getting a clean urine specimen for culture, and that means careful cleaning around the opening (penis in male and perineal area in the female) and a midstream collection which is then rapidly (within thirty minutes) examined in the laboratory. Sometimes the doctor will want to insert a needle into the bladder

in order to get a good specimen for examination and culture; while this is not routinely necessary, it is useful for someone with recurrent or more complicated infection problems.

2. *Sufficient treatment with an appropriate antibiotic:* This means a minimum of ten days of oral antibiotics or hospitalization for intravenous antibiotics in more serious cases.

3. *Rechecking urine cultures:* . . . two weeks and three months after an infection to make sure it has been completely eradicated.

None of these elements of treatment should be left out.

Any infection in a male and recurrent infections in the female merit further investigation for underlying causes. Such investigation should include an I.V.P. to check for anatomic defects that might cause infection to start. Infections are more likely in the female because of the proximity of the opening of the rectum and the vagina to the opening of the urinary tract; it is easy for "bugs" from the gut or the reproductive tract to get into the urinary tract. In the older population, infections are more common in the male, since enlarged prostates cause retention of urine, which promotes infection.

Improperly treated or unsuspected U.T.I.'s may lead to irreversible kidney damage, the development of hypertension, and other very serious problems. So it is important to aggressively diagnose and treat such infections. Chronic problems (recurrent infections, infections difficult to eradicate) must be thoroughly investigated by an appropriate specialist—nephrologist and/or urologist. The kidneys are too critical to take a chance on.

Sometimes it is tempting to ascribe urinary symptoms and blood in the urine (hematuria) to a "simple bladder infection"—acute hemorrhagic cystitis. This is indeed often the case in a female. But any such case should be investigated with cystoscopy and I.V.P. to rule out other causes of blood in the urine. Tumors of the urinary tract (see below) may be curable and should not be missed.

Kidney Stones

Stones may be found in any part of the urinary system— kidney, ureters, bladder. They most commonly produce the severe pain for which they are known when they pass down the ureters to the bladder. Stones in the kidney or bladder are less likely to produce such intense pain. Stones in any part of the urinary system may be associated with infection and produce correspondingly appropriate signs—fever, blood and/or pus in the urine, abdominal distress, urinary frequency, etc. Indeed, one of the reasons for investigating chronic or recurrent infections is to check for stones as an underlying cause.

The most common presenting situation for stones is the sudden onset of intense back and/or groin pain accompanied by nausea, sweating, and possibly bloody urine. Such a combination of symptoms is usually enough to bring the affected person to the hospital promptly, where examination, urinalysis, and an immediate I.V.P. will usually make the diagnosis without difficulty. The vast majority of stones will pass out of the urinary system spontaneously and will *not* require surgery; bed rest, fluids, and strong pain medicines for twenty-four to forty-eight hours will usually do the trick.

Once a diagnosis of a kidney stone has been made, it is essential to attempt to determine the composition of the stone and then institute any possible preventive program. Not all physicians are willing or able to engage in this "poststone" process. Certainly any person afflicted with recurrent stone formation should seek the advice of a "stone expert"—usually a urologist. Large teaching hospitals often have "stone clinics" for people with such problems; they might well be worth seeking out. The causes of stone formation are many and sometimes involve metabolic disease which must be corrected.

Tumors of the Urinary Tract

The key word in this section is hematuria—blood in the urine. *Hematuria must always be investigated,* even if it is intermittent or disappears. The hallmark of early tumors anywhere in the urinary system may be painless hematuria—without any other symptoms. This is one of the reasons that a microscopic exam of the urine should be done as part of any routine examination; some bleeding may be so minimal as to be seen only under the microscope.

Tumors of the urinary system vary considerably in growth and spread. For example, tumors of the bladder are often slow growing and may be excised through a tube inserted via the urethra—so-called "T.U.R." (transurethral resection). Tumors of the kidney, however, require more major surgery and removal of the entire affected kidney.

Again, any blood in the urine must be reported to your primary care physician. If you do not get satisfaction from him, seek the advice of a urologist.

Varicose Veins

Varicose veins of the lower leg are one of the more common afflictions of the human race. The veins involved are the superficial veins under the skin but outside the deep muscles of the leg; in this location, they are without much support and vulnerable to the increased pressure of standing and, in the female, of pregnancy. Aging and heredity are also thought to contribute to the weakening of these veins.

The most important point I can present in this book is the idea of preventing varicose veins by the use of support stockings, elastic stockings, leg exercising, *and* getting our legs up whenever we have the chance. (The person who props his or her legs up in the air whenever possible may not be socially acceptable but, medically speaking, well advised.) Such measures become especially important for the person with a strong family history of varicosities or for the person whose occupation requires continual standing. Once varicosities have occurred, further measures may be tried to prevent complications, such as skin changes which lead to skin ulcers. The idea, in other words, is not to pass off varicosities as something to accept as a part of life.

When varicosities become cosmetically and/or symptomatically significant, surgery (tying of veins and/or removing them) may be in order. One should not expect that surgery will cure all problems or that a recurrence will not be possible. But properly performed surgery can be very helpful in the very severe case. A general surgeon is the proper doctor to consult.

Venereal Disease

Venereal disease is "disease due to or propagated by sexual intercourse." There are five major forms of V.D. and several minor forms. In this country the two major forms of V.D. are still syphilis and gonorrhea, and I will confine my discussion to these two.

Before a more detailed discussion of each, I would like to make these general points:

1. The only certain prevention of V.D. is absolute and complete abstinence from sexual activity. *Anyone* engaging in sexual activity is at risk for V.D. Such a risk becomes less when sexual activity is confined to a mutually monogamous relationship—i.e., neither partner has sex with anyone else.

2. V.D. occurs only via the intimate contact of sexual activity—though insertion of the penis fully into the vagina is not required for contracting V.D. What is required is the direct contact of infected surfaces with other suitable surfaces—warm and moist. V.D. is *not* picked up from toilet seats, doorknobs, towels, etc.

3. There is currently no vaccine to protect against V.D. Having had V.D. does not make you immune; you can easily get reinfected.

4. The use of the condom will aid prevention but does not protect surfaces not separated by the condom. Various vaginal creams and foams used for contraceptive purposes *may* protect against V.D. "Morning-after" antibiotics can be useful but carry the risk of reactions to antibiotic injections.

Gonorrhea (GC) (Clap)

This disease is caused by a bacterium called *Neisseria gonorrhoeae,* a member of the gonococcal (hence the name GC) family of germs. GC has reached epidemic proportions in our society; in other words, it is every-where—among *all* classes, races, and ages.

The typical symptoms in men are painful and frequent urination plus a purulent (puslike) discharge from the penis; such symptoms occur anywhere from two days to weeks after exposure. Homosexual men may develop rectal and throat infection; GC must be suspected with symptoms in these areas. It used to be taught that men were always symptomatic and therefore would seek medical treatment. We now know that a significant percent of men infected with GC may have no symptoms and therefore be silent carriers.

Acute GC in the female may cause painful urination, vaginal discharge, and so on; such symptoms may be easily passed off as a urinary tract infection. Females may get throat infections from oral contact with an infected penis. Females are much more likely to be without symptoms than males—and therefore less likely to seek treatment. Also, the female is at greater risk for the spread of infec-tion to other parts of her anatomy—up into the womb and tubes—producing so-called P.I.D. (pelvic inflammatory disease). In both men and women, but more commonly in women, the GC germ may enter the blood stream, causing symptoms elsewhere—joints, heart, liver, brain, etc.

There is no simple blood test for the diagnosis of GC— a great drawback for detection and treatment. Diagnosis can only be made on the basis of specimens taken from infected locations which are then examined under the microscope and/or by culture (demonstrating growth in the lab). Slide tests are not adequate for the female; cultures are required and even these tests may not be accurate—in both males and females.

Appropriate doses of antibiotics (usually penicillin) will cure the vast majority of GC cases. Treatment is not the problem. Detection is.

Syphilis

Syphilis is caused by a germ named *Treponema pallidum*. It can enter the body through any moist, warm membrane or through an abrasion in the skin. Once in the body, the germ spreads and multiplies rapidly throughout the body. Four stages of the disease are possible:

1. The first sign of syphilis is the development of a sore called the "chancre" (pronounced "shanker"), usually at the site of entry—which is usually the genital area, though it may be anywhere entry occurred (fingers, lips, breast, anus, mouth, etc.). This "sore" is variable in appearance; it is usually painless. The sore will disappear whether or not treatment occurs. But if treatment does not occur, the germs continue to grow and multiply, leading to other possible stages.

2. Anywhere from a few weeks to many months later, the disease may manifest itself by rashes, joint pains, sore throat (and other symptoms similar to flu), etc. The symptoms are often suggestive of something else, and syphilis may never be thought of. During this time, the person infected may easily infect others via any kind of intimate contact—even kissing.

3. The next stage is called the latent stage. The disease may exist for many years without any symptoms—but the germs are still there.

4. This final stage is what kills people. Depending on where the germs have done their damage, the person may suffer and die from heart disease, brain destruction, etc.

There is one great "advantage" in having syphilis versus gonorrhea. Syphilis can be diagnosed by a blood test. Thousands of cases are detected every year by blood tests required for marriage, hospital admission, armed forces entry, etc. The only time a blood test is not valuable is in the very early stages of syphilis before the germ gets into the bloodstream. In the early stages, when only a sore is present, diagnosis must be made from samples of the sore looked at under the microscope. (Anyone suspected of gonorrhea should also have a blood test for syphilis since the two keep company.)

Treatment is, again, appropriate amounts of antibiotics—usually penicillin.

Summary

I have taken the time to describe these two diseases to give you a "feel" for their pervasiveness and seriousness. Now I would like to add a few words of practical advice:

1. Many private physicians are not equipped emotionally or otherwise to deal with V.D. Some physicians are very haphazard about the manner in which they test for and treat V.D. Also, some private physicians are not as careful as they should be about protecting confidentiality. Most states now provide free and confidential clinic services for the diagnosis and treatment of V.D.; your local or state health department should be able to provide a list of such facilities. In general,

these facilities are a better source of V.D. diagnosis and treatment than a private doctor.

2. Since V.D. diagnosis and treatment are often haphazard, it is *up to you* to ask for and insist on appropriate tests and treatment. *You* have a responsibility for checking out symptoms, for informing your sexual contact(s) when and if you are diagnosed with V.D., for insisting on screening tests as a part of any routine exams. I am not excusing the mistakes of the medical profession or the limited funds and effort devoted to V.D. by the government. But *you* are the one who will suffer from V.D.—not the profession or the government.

3. When you have been diagnosed and treated for V.D., it is *essential* that you arrange for followup tests to make sure that the disease has been eradicated.

Looking Ahead at American Health Care

The American Health Care Enterprise has no lack of analysts and I hesitate to add another voice to the fray. I certainly have no more right to speak than many others. But maybe because of circumstance I have a relatively neutral perspective that might be helpful.

I came into medicine from the ministry and from a family with no doctors and no encouragement to enter medicine; but, having come as a stranger, I have found a home in the world of medicine and the unique opportunity it provides to participate in human healing. I occupy a station in medicine (as an emergency-room physician) which happens to be, currently, the most conspicuous interface between consumer and provider, between the sick public unable to gain easy entry into health care and the harried professional trying to respond via traditional patterns. Also, as a public medical personality, I am constantly exposed to all sides of the great debate about the future of medical care. I identify with the anger of the sick public, but I also understand the concerns of the profession of which I am a part. It is from this middle ground that I wish to suggest three principles that must guide us all —public consumers, responsive government, concerned profession—as we attempt to heal the bitter hurts surrounding the healing art. These principles are: (1) health care is a right; (2) health care is costly; and (3) health care is personal.

I present these as so deceptively simple that we are likely to "move beyond" them quickly, but as so basic that to violate them at any stage of health care planning is to doom the result. I am deliberately avoiding a recital of horror stories, a detailed blueprint of correction. As in any great human endeavor, it is basic principles applied with consistency that we need—not more facts which we all know or can get intellectually but which we often cannot cope with creatively in the heat of emotion. So let's consider this a sermon in three parts from a minister who still has a strong streak of the preacher in him.

Health Care Is a Right

The enjoyment of the highest attainable standard of health is one of the fundamental rights of every human being without distinction of race, religion, political belief, economic or social condition. . . .
—PREAMBLE TO THE CONSTITUTION OF THE
WORLD HEALTH ORGANIZATION, JULY 1948

I present this first as being absolutely basic to any discussion concerning health care. Anyone who ignores those unable *for any reason* to obtain basic medical care ignores the fact that without health it becomes almost impossible to pursue life, liberty, or happiness. Emerson had these priorities in mind when he said that the *first* wealth of a nation is health. The sad truth now is that this wealthiest of nations is not the healthiest. We may get mad about the caricatured welfare recipient watching color TV in the back of a pink Cadillac, but that portrait *is* caricature. Reality consists of ignored children with rotten teeth, impoverished elderly citizens with cataracts, and unemployed families with no medical insurance.

At this point there is usually a protest from health professionals who say: Why pick on me? And there usually follows a recital of the very real wrongs in other areas of our public life—such as the incomprehensible waste of the military, the shenanigans of lawyers, the maneuverings of politicians, and on and on. And I agree that it is quite unfair to single out health care as the major symptom of what is really a national disease—namely, a consumptive greed loose in the land which so blinds the individual to our collective interdependence that a fine father accepts bribes when he puts on the police uniform, a loving husband encourages kickbacks when he puts on the political hat, and a wonderful neighbor encourages unnecessary and costly medical work when he dons the white coat.

But let me tell it like it is to my colleagues in health care. It does no good to moan about all the other inequities in American life. Health care professionals must accept the fact that love of health (and the omnipresent, suppressed fear of death) is paramount territory in the psyche of most people. The average citizen may get apoplectic about the crossed wires of Ma Bell or become red-faced about the indifference of General Motors; but let sickness touch his life and the king of all emotions—fear—takes center stage. And, as any student of nature knows, a fear-ridden animal is not to be underestimated. Politicians whose job it is to study the human animal know that health care is a very special concern for most people.

And let me hasten to prevent misunderstanding. I am not advocating, for example, requiring individual doctors to devote their entire professional lives to the care of people too poor to pay, too devoid of motivation (for whatever reason) to care about their own health, too full of hatred (for whatever reason) to provide the kind of gratitude that most of us need at least a small amount of. There are few like that—and I am not one of them. But I am saying that *all* of us in health care have got to get over that basic emotional hump so we can admit that health care (unlike the owning of a Cadillac) is a basic human right that must be provided if the society is capable of so doing. Having made this *moral* commitment, then we can begin to talk and plan *and* include ourselves in the talk and the plans—again, not total load but at least our fair share. Logistically this may require each health care professional and institution to participate in basic care—e.g., requiring professionals (whose training is increasingly subsidized by public money) to serve two years in medically deprived areas (in place of military service) and requiring all institutions (given licenses by the government to share in health profits) to also share in non-profit care.

Once we commit ourselves *nationally* to health care as a right, enormous implications follow. Probably the most basic implication is that the costs of basic health care should be removed from the *direct* responsibility of the individual and moved into the sector of public financing via tax revenues. The decisions as to what should be provided as *basic* will not be easy. Few would argue that treatment of heart failure qualifies as basic—but what about the straightening of crooked teeth—or noses? However, the ongoing debate about such questions should not keep us from getting at the now existent and basic but unmet medical needs of our citizens.

The example of public education is very appropriate. Having recognized education as a right, no sensible person would now advocate individual financial responsibility for the basic, elementary education of children; the thought of a father deciding, because of limited resources, which of his children learns to read strikes us as ridiculous. It is intriguing to determine the reasons for the acceptance of education as a right, while for so long denying health care the same legal and public status. It seems incredible that as recently as seven years ago the incoming president of the AMA could say in his inaugural speech: "It is not the right of the patient to be cared for by a physician but it is a privilege." It is interesting to speculate how long it will take for our courts and/or legislatures to give health care its rightful place in the gallery of unquestioned human rights.

Just as in education, however, a balance must be reached between publicly guaranteed services and private choices. Indeed, just as this country enters into this final phase of acknowledgment of health as a public right, we are, as a nation, questioning the monopolistic quality of public elementary education. But, while many are proposing the stimulating effect of private alternatives to public education, no one is suggesting that the financial responsibility for such basic education be returned to the private citizen.

Also, as in education, control should be local within broad federal guidelines that assure adequate basic and equal care to all. Undoubtedly court battles similar to the civil rights struggle in education will evolve, but they must be faced and won if this nation is to guarantee basic rights to all its citizens. However, there is no good evidence— and increasingly much to the contrary—that a large federal bureaucracy is successful at actually running anything that requires sensitivity to individual needs and situations. Federally enforced guidelines, yes; but central administration, no.

Finally, just as in education, opportunities can be provided but any significant result requires effort on the part of the recipient. The man who decries the high cost of medical care while smoking three packs a day is similar to the citizen who complains about the cost of energy while guzzling gas at 75 m.p.h. The person who waits until a crisis arises before seeking medical care is similar to the student who starts the term paper the night before it is due. Half the hospitalizations in this country are for diseases of the cardiovascular system, injuries due to accidents, respiratory diseases, and mental illness. Much of such hospitalization is needless—the result of people imposing risks on themselves.

In short, I am suggesting that public education provides a useful model, though obviously it cannot be applied in total detail. I believe that such policies will be of benefit to the public. I also believe that such policies will ultimately prove beneficial to the medical profession—though not necessarily financially. By removing the financial burden directly from the individual and freeing the doctor from remunerative considerations in relation to any given patient, the air now surrounding the healing encounter between patient and doctor should be cleared of much bitterness. (I will also suggest that this kind of policy could be applied to all "service professions" which have become a necessity in modern life—including lawyers, plumbers, and car mechanics.) I am well aware that this sounds very socialistic—which is far from my intention; and I must add that a ruthless disregard for any minority—including a professional one—ultimately weakens all of a democracy. But *any* system of government, including democracy, fails in my estimation if it cannot provide basic health care for all its citizens.

Health Care Is Costly

Once we commit ourselves as a nation to health care as a right, we must be willing as a nation to pay the cost, *whatever it is.* Given the fact that health care is now approaching ten percent of our GNP, such a commitment may boil down to the "butter versus guns" choice—so I go on record as favoring butter (or at least polyunsaturated margarine). And I will become even more simplistic: All the talk about which health plan costs the most is irrelevant. Having determined what is needed and what the most productive method(s) are of meeting these needs, we as a nation must pay the bill—confident that it will be money at least as well spent as those millions spent on aircraft never used and now lying low on Arizona sands. And the bill will inevitably include correction of social ills that account for so much ill health.

One other observation about emotions is in order. The intrusion of sickness into our lives is just that—an intrusion. Illness is not requested, and it defies our sense of justice to have to pay for something we didn't ask for (though we all know that many times illness is the result of the way we choose to live). We may grumble about high prices and high taxes, but we have at least some sense of receiving in return something we want or need. But not so with sickness—which is annoying at least and devastating at worst. And to have to pay—sometimes at extreme sacrifice—for this uninvited villain is the final insult. This is something that we physicians, who often do not have to pay for health care, cannot appreciate.

Let me again comment briefly on the emotional issue of physician incomes, reminding you that such is a small part of our total health expenditure. I defend the propriety of physicians earning a very good income. Since we have not yet attained the heavenly state (where money is reportedly viewed as an illicit love affair), we have to be earthly and realistic and recognize money for what it is —the way our society attempts to reward. Given the investment of training time, working time, and emotional responsibility, most doctors are entitled to a very good reward. (Not many people will dispute this as a theory; as suggested before it's their own bill that gripes them.) Of course I cannot defend the greedy physician with high income who provides minimal service. (Indeed, this principle of the honest earning of income, if applied rigorously to all areas of our national life, would result in unbelievable consternation—witness the high income of lucky birth and low income of teachers to whom we entrust our children for so much of their formative years.) And I am very concerned about the trend of physicians to seek comfortable subspecialty positions with high fees for piecemeal work while crying needs in primary care are ignored. But again I defend the earnings of the majority of physicians as being at least as legitimate as most other earnings in our society. We must always expect to pay a fair price for quality medical care; it can never be free.

A commitment to basic health care as a right for all will be costly in other ways than just money. For physicians it will be costly in terms of traditional independence as increasing peer review and some form of placement in areas of need become inevitable. For hospitals it will be costly in terms of submission of parochial pride to regional needs. For drug and scientific industries it will be costly in terms of increasing scrutiny of profits and priorities. For some of our citizens it will be costly in terms of the "haves" curtailing nonessential demands and sharing initially limited resources with the "have-nots." And for the nation it will be costly in terms of a basic attack on the social ills responsible for so much of our ill health—highway accidents secondary to drinking and speeding; lung cancer secondary to incredible hypocrisy in government and the tobacco industry; the rats and malnutrition and lead poisoning of ghetto investment. Indeed, one must conclude that our political leaders do not really care about improved health per se as long as they simply talk about changes in health care and ignore relatively simple (but politically painful) solutions which could improve the health of the nation, comparatively speaking, overnight.

Health Care Is Personal

Since the original New Deal days the answer of American society to social problems has been to "let the government do it." All of us deal daily with big government—from standing in line at the Driver's License Bureau to driving on a bridge in a state of perpetual repair—and we grumble about it but manage to survive. I am not out to engage in diatribe against the government—which, after all, consists of human beings like us. I am, however, extremely worried that the personal touch may also be increasingly lost where it may be most essential: in the healing encounter.

It is popular to castigate medicine as a "cottage industry"; it is easy to minimize the traditional one-to-one relationship of patient and doctor—as long as you are a politician who knows he can call *his* personal physician when illness strikes. And I welcome the application of efficiency techniques and management expertise to the practice of medicine. But I must raise the flag of caution to make sure that apparent gains are not offset by immeasurable losses. I shudder to think of physicians who no longer worry about their patients after five o'clock because someone else is "taking over," physicians who no longer have the incentive to do their best because a massive system cares little about such things as compassion and reliability, physicians who have forgotten how to give of themselves because the feedback consists only of impersonal printouts and administrative directives.

Despite material affluence in this country, our human spirit gives evidence of poverty. And this kind of deprivation takes its toll: the harried executive on the climb whose innards grind out GI pains, the lonely housewife whose heartaches translate into headaches. These people will receive standard and accepted treatment; gas pills and pain pills. But real healing may require the kind of encounter that is so difficult to find these days: a relationship with someone who simply cares—not only with professional sophistication but with a personal touch. As we sit at the drawing boards and design sweeping changes in health care, we must be careful not to blueprint out the possibility for this type of encounter within the walls of the healing arts—or we will all be left with a dry bone where we sought the sustenance of healing.

I wish to close this section (and the book) by quoting some words from Albert Schweitzer which I carry on the inside leaf of my daily appointment book. I find them, each time I read them, a useful reminder. And I suggest that they apply to all of us—professional and nonprofessional, as we seek healing in these times.

But to everyone, in whatever state of life he finds himself, the ethics of reverence for life do this: they force him without cessation to be concerned at heart with all the human destinies and all the other life-destinies which are going through their life-course around him, and to give himself as man, to the man who needs a fellow-man. They will not allow the scholar to live only for his learning, even if his learning makes him very useful, nor the artist to live only for his art, even if by means of it he gives something to many. They do not allow the very busy man to think that with his professional activities he has fulfilled every demand upon him. They demand from all that they devote a portion of their life to their fellows.

Bibliography

The following suggestions represent standard medical sources of information. I offer them in the confidence that most persons with basic intelligence and genuine interest should be able to understand such material (with the help of a good medical dictionary such as Dorland's). At the very least, the reading of such material will prepare you for a more intelligent dialogue with your sources of medical care.

1. *Harrison's Principles of Internal Medicine* (Wintrobe et al.; McGraw-Hill). This classic (originally edited by Dr. Harrison and still referred to as "Harrison's") is the standard American textbook on internal medicine. It is large and expensive, but often available in good general libraries and in all medical libraries. The book is generally quite readable and offers a fair summary of most important questions in adult medicine. I recommend it as a general starting point for most adult medical problems. Since the book is not a surgical text, it often is brief on the subject

of surgery; on the other hand, its surgical views are often more detached than one might find in a surgical text.

2. *Principles of Surgery* (Schwartz et al.; McGraw-Hill). A relative newcomer to the list of standard surgical texts, this book is widely regarded as a source of sound, modern surgical information. Important surgical problems receive extensive discussion as to the indications for doing surgery —which is the particular issue that most lay persons would be interested in.

3. *Gynecology Principles and Practice* (Kistner; Year Book Medical Publishers). This is a very readable medical book packed full of good information. Entirely written by Dr. Kistner, a well-known Harvard gynecologist, the book has a consistency of style often missing in larger, edited works.

4. *Textbook of Pediatrics* (Nelson et al.; Saunders). Usually referred to as Nelson's Textbook, this classic and standard book is scheduled for a new edition this year.

I offer the above four books as excellent sources of information in the four basic primary care areas. There are many other first-rate medical books, but these suggestions offer a start. In addition, the Lange Medical Publications of Los Altos, California, offer a series of relatively low-cost textbooks (in paperback form) in all of the major primary care and specialty fields. Briefer, and providing more of a summary, these texts are more difficult to read without a good medical background, but they are sources of standard information. *Current Medical Diagnosis and Treatment* is offered for $12 and a new edition appears each year; this text might serve as a handy reference for the person with ongoing medical questions and interests.

I remind you again of the many excellent sources of lay information available in the popular media. As suggested earlier, at the very least these discussions alert you to some of the controversial issues in medicine today. There are also many good lay medical encyclopedias which attempt to offer a comprehensive discussion of most major medical problems. Two of the better ones are *Ladies' Home Journal Family Medical Guide* (Nourse; Harper & Row) and *The Complete Medical Guide* (Miller; Simon & Schuster).

Finally, I would remind you of two books mentioned in my discussions of Women's Health Problems and Nutrition.

1. *Our Bodies, Ourselves: A Book By and For Women* (by the Boston Women's Health Book Collective; Simon & Schuster). This inexpensive paperback is strong on both opinion and good information. While I don't agree with some of it, I do think it represents a unique effort to bring together information not readily available elsewhere —particularly in such areas as sexuality and the problems of the female in obtaining health care. The sections on obstetrical care are excellent.

2. *The Family Guide to Better Food and Better Health* (Deutsch; Bantam Books). This low-cost paperback covers all of the important topics in nutrition in a fair yet informative manner.

Index

Abdomen, examination of, 160, 163
  appendicitis, 163
  GI diseases, 160
  pain, 336
  surgery, 219–220
Abortions, 299, 333
  following exposure to rubella, 301–302
Acid-base disturbances, 28
Acidosis, 143
Acne, severe, 349
Acupuncture, 241–242
Adenoids and adenoidectomies, 369–370
Air pollution, effect on lung disease, 145
Alcoholism, 149, 178–180
  effect on liver, 178–179
    cirrhosis, 179
    hepatitis, 178–179
  incidence of cancer and, 179
Allergists, 21–22, 244–245
  life-threatening emergencies, 243
  reactions, 241–243
Allied health personnel, 40
Alopecia (baldness), 258–259
American Academy of Family Physicians, 25, 40
American Academy of General Practice, 25
American Academy of Orthopedic Surgeons, 257
American Board of Family Practice, 26
American Cancer Society, 153
  Reach to Recovery program, 230–231
American College of Emergency Physicians, 37
American Diabetes Association, 314
American Heart Association, 88

American Medical Association, 199, 314
Amino acids, 198, 201–202
  deficiency in children, 202
Amniocentesis, 239, 333
  role in genetic counseling, 288–289
Anaphylactic shock, 243
Androgens, 238
Anemias, 137–138, 245–247
  diagnosis and treatment, 246–247
  headaches and, 304
  iron-deficiency, 206, 246–247
  pernicious, 206
  sickle-cell, 343
  types and causes, 246
Anesthesia, administration of, 56
Anesthesiologists, 13, 36, 56
Anesthetists, 56
Aneurysms, congenital, 359
Angiography, cerebral, 361
Annual physical examinations, 67–69
  (*See also* Physical examinations)
Antacids, use of, 181
Antibiotics, 77
  hypersensitivity reaction in liver, 177
  for infectious diseases, 187–190
  for local infections, 191–192
  in high-risk patients, 192
  for strep throat, 133–134, 356–357
  (*See also* under name of disease)
Antibodies, 152–153
Anticholinergic drugs, 337
Anticoagulant drugs, 360–361
  for thrombophlebitis, 366
Antigens, 242
Antihistamines, 244, 337
Antispasmodic drugs, 181

Anxiety of patients, 77–78
Appendicitis, 163–164
Arrhythmias, 124, 126
Arteriosclerosis, 119
Arthritis, 28, 247–251
  of the back, 253–254
  "fad" or "quack" cures, 250
    copper bracelets, 250
  osteoarthritis, 253
  rheumatoid, 247–248, 253
  sickle-cell abnormalities and, 343
  of the spine, 254
  surgical procedures, 248–250
    knee replacements, 250
    "total hip replacement," 248–250
  treatment, 248–251
Arthrography, 105
Aspirin, 185
  irritant effect of, 180, 295, 332
  long-term anticoagulation, 366
Asthma, 251–252
  emotional component in, 251–252
Atherosclerosis ("hardening of the arteries"), 116, 237
  coronary artery disease, 119–121
  diabetes and, 278–279
  hypertension and, 310–311
  stroke prevention and, 359–361
  thrombosis and, 358
Audiologists, 281
Australian antigen, 176
Autopsies, 36

Back pain, 252–258
  arthritis, 253–254
  congenital deformities, 254
  disk disease, 254–257
  low-back pain, 32, 252
    doctors, 257–258
  muscle strain, 252–253
Bad breath (halitosis), 184
Balanced diets, 198–200
  (*See also* Diet and nutrition)
Baldness (alopecia), 258–259
  hair transplants, 258–259
Barbiturate medications, 288
Barium x-ray studies, 161, 165–166, 306

Bed-wetting (enuresis), 259–260
Bibliography, 401–403
Biopsies, 27
  breast cancer, 227–228
  prostate gland, 340
Birth control, 260–270
  (*See also* Contraception)
Birth-control pills, 262–267
  adverse effects, 263, 265–266
  birth defects and, 265
  blood clot formation and, 264–265, 364
  cancer and, 263–264
  during first three months of pregnancy, 332–333
  effect on subsequent fertility, 265–266
  estrogen content, 266
  "mini-pill" and "morning after" pill, 266
Black people: risk of hypertension, 309
  sickle-cell abnormalities, 297–298, 343–344
  screening tests, 344–345
Bladder disorders, 35
  infections, 376–377
  stones, 377–378
  tumors, 378
  (*See also* Urinary tract problems)
Bleeding problems, 92–93
  application of direct pressure, 92–93
  female, 215–216, 234
    postmenopausal, 216, 234, 238
    premenopausal, 216
  gastrointestinal, 162, 184–185
    life-threatening emergency, 184
    warning signs, 184–185
  massive bleeding, 92–93
  from rectum, 165
Blood: diseases, 27
  GI bleeding, 162, 184–185
  massive bleeding, 92–93
  in urine (hematuria), 376–378
Blood clot formation: birth control pills and, 264–265, 364
  cerebral thrombosis, 358
  to the lung (pulmonary emboli), **94, 367–368**

thrombophlebitis, 362–368
Blood counts, 304
Blood fats, risk factor in heart
    disease, 130–131
Blood pressure, periodic checkups,
    68
Blood sugar checks, 69
    (*See also* Diabetes)
Blood tests, 36
    for cholesterol and triglycerides,
    69, 130–131
Blood transfusions and hepatitis,
    176
Board certified doctors, 16
    "board eligible," 16
Body temperature, rectal and oral,
    294–295
Boils and carbuncles, 350–351
    I & D (incision and drainage),
    351
Bone and joint problems, 31–32
    simple fractures, 31–32
Boston Women's Health Book
    Collective:
    Our Bodies, Ourselves, 326, 329,
    335
Bowel diseases: cancer, 152
    constipation, 182–183
    inflammatory, 172–174
    investigation of persistent
        changes in normal habits,
        162–164, 182–183
Brain damage: due to lack of
    oxygen, 88–89
    minimal, 307
    strokes, 357
    techniques for diagnosing, 99–100
Brain disorders, 29
    significance of seizures, 342
Brain scans, 304
Brain tumors, 29
Brain wave studies, 342
Breast cancer, 30, 152, 221–231
    diagnosis and treatment, 226–227
    biopsies, 227–228
    early detection, 68, 154, 223–226
    mammography, 225
    monthly self-examination, 68,
        223–225

physical examination by doctor,
    225
    thermography, 226
    mammary dysplasia ("lumpy
        breasts"), 222–223
    risk factors, 221–223
    surgical treatment, 228–229
    localized operations, 228
    postsurgical treatment, 230–231
    psychological impact, 228, 230–
        231
    radical surgery, 228–229
Breast feeding, 324, 334–335
Breathing problems, 86–88
    acute, 28
    cardiopulmonary resuscitation,
        87–88
    life-threatening emergencies,
        86–87
    role of anesthesiologists, 36
Bronchiectasis, 144
Bronchioles (air passages), 144
Bronchitis (chronic lung disease),
    141, 143–146, 191
    acute, 144
    flu shots, 193
Bruises, 362–363
Burns, 101–104
    control of pain, 103
    degree of burn, 101–103
        first-degree, 102
        second-degree, 102–103
        third-degree, 103
    emergency treatment, 101–104
        cold applications, 102
        skin grafting, 54, 103–104
        sterile dressings, 102
    inhalation of hot gases or flames,
        103
    intravenous fluids, 103
    therapy, 103–104
    plastic surgery, 54, 103–104

Caffeine and coffee drinking, 132,
    138, 180–181
Calcium, need for, 207–208
Calories, 196–198
Cancer, 151–157
    birth-control pills and, 263–264
    of blood cells, 27

Cancer (*cont.*)
  breast (*see* Breast cancer)
  causes, 153–154
    carcinogenic chemicals, 154
    chronic irritation, 154
    smoking, 154–155
    viruses, 154
  cervical, 220, 231–234
  curable, 152
  diagnosis and treatment, 151–157
    choosing a doctor, 156–157
    sources of information, 156–157
  early detection, 153–154
  endometrial, 233, 235
  familial tendencies, 153–154
  GI tract, 162
  hospital expertise, 156–157
    tumor committee, 156–157
  immunology, 152–153
    use of tuberculosis vaccine
      (BGG), 153
  leukemias, 27
  lung, 147–148
  Pap smears, 233
  of prostate gland, 340
  radial neck surgery, 32
  skin, 351–352
  stomach, 152
  thyroid gland, 371
  treatment, 154–155
    radiation therapy, 155
    surgery, 32, 155
  tumors, benign, 152
    malignant, 152
  uterine and cervical, 231–234,
    264
  "vaginal," 264
  warning signs, 153–154
Carbohydrates, 200–201
Carbon tetrachloride, hypersensitivity reactions, 177, 375
Carbuncles and boils, 350–351
Cardiac surgeons, 34
Cardiologists, 15, 117, 139
Cardiology (diseases of heart), 26
  pediatric, 32
**Cardiopulmonary resuscitation
(CPR), 87–88
instructions, 88**

CAT (Computerized Axial Tomography), 100
Cataracts, 291–293
  surgery, 291–293
Cerebral angiography, 99, 304
Cerebral embolism, 358
Cerebrovascular accidents (CVA's),
  94, 311, 357–362
  (*See also* Strokes)
Cerumen (ear wax), 283–284
Cervicitis, 220
Cervix, cancer of, 152, 220, 231–234
  cause and risk, 232
  diagnosis and screening, 232–234
    Pap smears, 233
  treatment, 235–236
Chemotherapy, 155
Chest, rib injuries, 112–113
Chest pains, 117–119
  heart disease and, 117–119
  **life-threatening emergencies,
    118–119**
  sources of, 117–118
Chest surgeons, 34
Chest X-rays, 69
  for tuberculosis, 148–150
Childbirth, natural, 328–329
Children and infants:
  heart disease, 116
  immunization shots, 109
  nutrition, 202
Chiropractors, 38
Choking, 89–92
  **attempt to retrieve material,
    90–91**
  blockage of windpipe, 89–90
  Heimlich maneuver, 91–92
  **opening air passage in windpipe,
    92**
  small child, 90
Cholecystectomy, 169
Cholecystitis (inflammation of gall
  bladder), 168
Choledocholithiasis (stones in duct
  system), 168
Cholelithiasis (stone in gall bladder), 168
Cholesterol, 69, 131, 203
  heart disease and, 130–131

Choosing a doctor, 47–49
  age of physician, 49
  for allergy problems, 244–245
  for cancer, 156–157
  for ear problems, 279–280
  geographical convenience, 48
  getting inside information,
    48
  heart specialists, 117
  hospital affiliation, 7, 17, 47–48
  peer review, 47, 396
  physician's training and ex-
    pertise, 48
  shopping around, 48
  for skin problems, 348–349
  when moving to a new place, 49
  for urinary tract problems, 373
  (*See also* Physicians)
Cigarette smoking (*see* Smoking)
Circulation:
  collapsed person, 86–87
  feeling for pulse, 86–87
  need for cardiopulmonary re-
    suscitation, 87–88
Cirrhosis of the liver, 177–178
  alcoholic, 177–179
  causes and treatment, 177–178
Clinical information, 80
  randomized clinical trials, 80
Clinics, 44–45
  "free clinic" movement, 44
  group practice, 44–45
  primary care functions, 41, 81
Clomiphene (Clomid), 266, 319
Coffee drinking, excessive, 132, 138,
  180–181
Colds (*See* Common colds)
Colitis, 173–174
Colon: cancers, 162, 164–166, 231
  diagnosis, 185
  Crohn's disease, 173
  diet and, 165–166
  "irritable colon syndrome," 173–
    174
  polyps, 165
  ulcerative colitis, 173
Colostomies, 166
"Common cold," 187–195
  antibiotics for, 187–190

bacterial and viral infections,
  187–189
flu shots, 192–193
treatment, 194
upper respiratory infections, 190–
  191
use of vitamin C, 192
Computerized Axial Tomography
  (CAT), 100
Congestive heart failure, 134–137
Constipation, 182–183
Contraception (birth control), 260–
  270
  artificial insemination, 262
  birth control pills, 262–267
  condoms and jellies, 268–269
  diaphragms and jellies, 268
  foam and jellies alone, 268
  hormonal suppression of ovula-
    tion, 262–267
  injectable hormone contracep-
    tion, 266
  IUD's (intrauterine devices), 267–
    268
  need for seeking sound counsel,
    269–270
  rhythm method, 269
  sterilization procedures, 261–262
    tubal ligation in females, 261
    vasectomies in males, 261
Coronary angiography, 122–124
  risks involved, 123
Coronary artery disease, 116, 119–
  132
  atherosclerosis process, 119–121,
    129
  bypass surgery, 124–125
  cause of heart failure, 135
  coronary angiography, 122–124
  diagnosis, 122–124
  nation's No. 1 health problem,
    116, 132
  obesity and, 323
  treatment, 124–128
    bypass surgery, 124–125
    medical treatment, 124
  warning signs, 121
Coronary care units, 126–127
Cromolyn sodium, 252

Counterpulsation devices, 127–128
CPR (*see* Cardiopulmonary resuscitation)
Crohn's disease of the colon, 173
Cuts (*see* Lacerations)
CVA's (cerebrovascular accidents) (*see* Strokes)
Cystocele, 217
Cystoscopy, urinary tract problems, 373

D & C (dilation and curettage) 215–216, 233–234
Dalkon Shield (IUD), 267
Dental care, 270–272
  adult tooth care, 271–272
  fluorides, 271
  periodontal disease, 24, 272
  preserving "baby teeth," 271
Dentists, 22–24
Depo-Provera (injectable hormone contraception), 266
Depression, mental, 284
  (*See also* Emotional disorders)
Dermatologists, 24–25, 259, 348
DES (diethystilbestrol), 264, 266
Deutsch, Ronald M., 195, 199
Diabetes, 27, 149, 272–279
  in adults, 273–275
  avoidance of birth-control pills, 265
  in children, 273–276
  complications, 273, 278–279
    from excessive swings in blood sugar, 278
    eye diseases, 278–279
    kidney diseases, 278–279
    premature atherosclerosis, 278–279
  diagnosis, 273–275
    blood sugar tests, 69, 273–274
    glucose tolerance tests (GTT), 274, 313
    "urine screening," 273
  disorders of glucose metabolism, 273
  infections, 278
    foot care, 278
  insulin deficiency, 273, 275–276

obesity and, 278, 324
risk factor in heart disease, 130, 278–279
symptoms, 275–276
treatment, 275–278
  diet and weight loss, 276–278, 324
  exercise, 277–278
  insulin, 275–276
  "juvenile diabetics," 275
  oral drugs, 276–277
Diagnosticians, 27
Diet and nutrition, 194–209
  balance in, 198–200
  basic food groups, 199
  calcium, 207–208
  calories, 196–198
  carbohydrates, 200–201
  colon cancer, 165–166
  disease cures, 208–209
  during pregnancy, 331–332
  effect of exercise, 197
  essential nutrients, 198
  fats, 203–204
  fluorides, 208
  health foods, 206–207
    organic foods, 207
  iron, 208
  lecithin, 208
  MDR (minimal daily requirement) lists, 199
  obesity treatments, 325
  proteins, 201–202
  RDA (recommended daily allowance), 198–199
  safe and effective, 209
  salt intake, 208, 312
  treatment of ulcers, 181
  vitamins, 204–206
Diethylstilbestrol (DES), 264, 266
Digestive difficulties, 27, 159–185
  gall bladder disease, 168, 170
  (*See also* Gastrointestinal diseases)
Digitalis, 136
  toxicity, 136
Dilation and curettage (D&C), 215–216, 233–234
Diphtheria, pertussis and tetanus (DPT) shots, 109

Directory of Medical Specialists, The, 17
Disabled persons, maintenance care, 71
Discograms, 255
Disk disease, 254–257
  cause of back pain, 254–257
  injections of chymopapain, 256–257
  surgery for, 32, 256–257
Diuretics ("water-pills"), 136–137
Diverticulosis and diverticulitis, 166–167
  endoscopic exam, 167
  exploratory surgery, 167
  treatment and diet, 167
Down's syndrome (mongolism), 296, 299, 333
DPT shots (diphtheria, pertussis and tetanus), 109
Drowsiness following head injury, 97–98
Drugs: allergic reactions, 242–243
  barbiturate medications, 288
  cancer therapy, 155
  for emotional illness, 287–289
  hypersensitivity reactions in liver, 176–177
  lithium, 288
  tranquilizers, 287–288
  stimulants, effect on hyperactive children, 307–308
Dyspareunia, 221

Ear problems, 279–284
  choosing a doctor, 279–280
  ear infections, 187, 279, 281–283
    accumulation of fluid, 283
    antibiotics and antihistamines, 282–283
    mastoid infection, 283
    middle ear, 282–283
    otitis externa, 282
    treatment, 282–283
  ear wax (cerumen), 283–284
  earaches, 282
  hearing loss, 279
    acoustic neuroma, 281
    conductive and sensorineural, 280–281

  hearing aids, 281
    prevention of, 281
    surgical treatment, 281
  injury to ear, 281
  noise pollution and, 282
Edema, pulmonary, 136
Education, everyone's right to public, 390–391
Educational programs: continuing education for doctors, 17–19
  for hospital staffs, 11
Electrical injuries, emergency care, 93
Electrocardiograms (ECG), 69, 122
Electroencephalograms (EEG), 304, 342
Electrolyte imbalance, 28
Emboli (blood clot), 363, 365
  cerebral, 358
  pulmonary, 94, 367–368
Emergencies, 70, 85–114
  bleeding, massive, 92–93
  breathing and circulation difficulties, 86–87
  burns, 101–104
  cardiopulmonary resuscitation (CPR), 87–88, 93
  choking, 89–92
  "collapse" situations, 85–96
    cardiopulmonary resuscitation, 87–88
    causes of collapse, 88–96
    circulation and breathing difficulties, 86–87
    life-threatening situations, 89–96
  electrical injury, 93
  eye injuries, 101, 290
  fainting, 95
  frostbite, 114
  head injuries, 96–100
  heart attacks, 89
  heatstroke, 113
  joint injuries, 104–106
  lacerations (cuts), 106–110
  massive blood clot to the lung (pulmonary emboli), 94, 367–368
  near-drowning, 94
  nosebleeds (epistaxis), 110–111

Emergencies (cont.)
  poisoning, 100–101
  rib injury, 112–113
  seizures, 95
  shock, 95–96
  stroke ("cerebrovascular acci-
    dents"), 94, 357–362
  sudden unconsciousness, 88–89
  syncope (fainting), 95
Emergency room physicians, 36–37,
  389
Emotional illness, 138–139, 284–
  289
  diagnosis, 284–286
  hallucinations, 284
  inability to function, 285–286
  manifestations of, 284–286
  mental health clinics, 286–287
  psychiatrists, 15, 33, 286
  psychotherapy and, 288–289
  recognizing, 284–286
  treatment, 286–289
    choice of doctors, 33, 286–287
    drugs or shock therapy, 287–
    289
Emphysema (chronic lung disease),
  28, 143–146
  causes, 143
  effect of smoking, 145, 354
  flu shots, 193
  protein deficiency, 144
  screening programs, 144
  symptoms, 143
  treatment, 144–146
Endocrine Society, 314
Endocrinologists, 27, 314
Endocrinology (diseases of endocrine glands), 26–27, 32
Endodontists, 22–23
Endometriosis, 217
Endoscopy, 27, 161, 167
Eneuresis (bed-wetting), 259–260
ENT (Ear, Nose and Throat)
  specialists, 32, 280
  for sinus infections, 347
Epilepsy, 340–342
  discrimination against epileptics,
    342
  drug control of, 341–342

emergency reactions to seizures,
  341
  significance of seizures, 341–342
Esophagus: cancer, 152, 162
  reflux esophagitis, 170–171
  source of chest pain, 118
  thoracic surgery, 34
Estrogen-deficiency problems, 236–
  238
Exercise: effect on weight loss, 197,
  325–326
  heart disease and, 131–132
Eye problems, 289–294
  cataracts, 291–293
  choosing a doctor, 30–32
    ophthalmologists, 30–31
  diabetes and, 278–279
  emergencies, 290
  glaucoma, 31, 293–294
  medications, 291
  "pink eye" (viral conjunctivitis),
    291
  symptoms, 290–291
  treatment for poisons in eye, 101

Facial injuries, 35
  plastic surgery, 54–55
FACS (Fellow of the American
  College of Surgeons), 16
"Fad" or "quack" cures for arthritis, 250
Fainting spells, emergency treatment, 95
Family Guide to Better Food and
  Better Health, The (Deutsch),
  195, 199
Family physician movement, 25–26
  certifying exams, 26
  primary care functions, 40–41, 81
  recertification requirements, 18
  training programs, 40
Family planning, 269
Fatigue, problems of, 246
Fats, blood (hyperlipidemias), 130–
  131
  polyunsaturated, 131
  risk factor in heart disease, 130–
    131
Fats in diet, 198, 203–204

saturated and unsaturated, 203
Fees and fee schedules, 59–65
  attitudes of public, 59–60, 393–394
  doctor-in-training, 60
  fee disputes and fee gouging, 64–65
  fee-for-services vs. salary, 63–64
  hospital-based physicians, 63
  inequities among various specialties, 61–62
  need for financial incentive, 63–64
  schedules, 62–63
    established by third parties, 62
  surgical procedures, 55, 61–62
Fetal monitoring and care, 333–334
  (*See also* Obstetrical care)
Fevers, 28, 294–295
  aspirin and rest for, 295
  body temperature and, 294–295
  symptoms, 28, 294–295
Fibroids (benign tumors of the uterus), 216–217, 264
Fisher, Dr. Bernard, 228
Flatulence (gas), GI symptom, 183
Flu syndrome, 191
  value of "flu shots," 192–193
Fluorides in drinking water, 208, 271
Food and Drug Administration, 198–199, 257, 266–267, 277
Ford, Mrs. Betty, 228
Framingham (Mass.) study of risk factors in heart disease, 128
Frostbite, emergency treatment, 114
FUO's (fevers of unknown origin), 28
Furuncles, 350–351

Gall bladder disease, 168–170
  cancer, 162
  cholecystitis (inflammation of gall bladder), 168
  choledocholithiasis (stones in duct system), 168
  cholelithiasis (stones in gall bladder), 168
  function of gall bladder, 168
  surgery, 169
  treatment with pills to "dissolve" gallstones, 169–170
Gamma globulin for hepatitis, 176
"Gastritis," diagnosis of, 174
Gastroenteritis: transient, 164
  viral, 162, 174
Gastroenterologists, 159, 172
Gastroenterology, 27
Gastrointestinal (GI) diseases, 159–185
  "acute abdomen," 160
  appendicitis, 163–164
  cancers of GI tract, 162
    of colon and rectum, 164–166
    early diagnosis important, 185
  diagnosis, 159–161
    barium X-rays, 161
    endoscopy, 161
    sigmoidoscopy, 161
    X-ray studies, 161
  diet and nutrition, 165–166
  diverticulosis and diverticulitis, 166–167
  gall bladder disease, 168–170
  gastroenterologists, 159, 172
  GI system, 159–160
  heartburn (reflux esophagitis) and hiatus hernia, 170–172
  inflammatory bowel disease, 172–174
  liver disease, 175–179
  medical specialists, 159–160
  physical examinations, 160
  surgery, 160
  symptoms, 162, 182–185
    constipation, 182–183
    diarrhea, 162
    flatulence (gas), 183
    gastrointestinal bleeding, 184–185
    halitosis (bad breath), 184
    nausea, 162
    vomiting, 162
  ulcers, 179–182
  viral infections, 162, 174
  "wait and see" attitude, 160
  withholding of pain medications, 160

Gastrointestinal (GI) diseases (cont.)
X-ray studies, 161
General Practitioners (GP), 15, 25–
26
family physician movement, 25–
26
primary care role, 39, 81
(See also Primary care physicians)
Genetic counseling, 296–298
for prospective parents, 298
role of amniocentesis, 288–289
sickle-cell abnormalities, 343
techniques, 297–298
diagnosis of past problems, 297
family history, 297
screening studies, 297–298
trained personnel for, 297
German measles (rubella), 300–302
abortions for pregnant women,
301–302
blood tests for, 300–301
problem of exposure in pregnant
women, 301–302, 317
rubella vaccine, 300–302, 316–317
GI series, 36
(See also Gastrointestinal diseases)
Glaucoma, 181, 293–294
testing for, 31, 68, 293–294
Glomerulonephritis, 374–375
antecedent strep infection, 374–
375
Glucose tolerance tests (GTT),
274, 313
Gonorrhea (clap), 380–382
diagnosis and treatment, 381–382
symptoms, 381–382
GP (see General practitioners)
Group practice, 43–46
clinics, 44–45
HMO's (Health Maintenance
Organizations), 45–46
partnership arrangements, 44
Gynecologists, 29–30, 212–213
cancer expertise, 156
infertility problems, 218
urinary tract problems, 373
Gynecology, 29–30

Hair loss, 258–259
baldness, 258–259

hair transplants, 258–259
Halitosis (bad breath), 184
Hallucinations, 284
Hands, plastic surgery, 54
"Hardening of the arteries" (see
Atherosclerosis)
Harvard Medical School, Department of Continuing Educa-
tion, 19
Hay fever, 21, 244
Head injuries, 29
children, 96–98
drowsiness, headaches and vomiting following, 97–98
emergency treatment, 96–100
medical evaluation, 98–99
cerebral angiography, 99
skull X-rays, 98–99
posttraumatic syndrome, 99
unconscious patient, 96–97
Headaches, 29, 302–305
aspirin for, 302–303
choosing a doctor, 304–305
cluster, 303–304
following head injury, 97–98
"Horton's or "histamine," 303–304
life-threatening emergencies, 302
migraine, 303–304
"tension," 302
tests ("headache workup"), 304–
305
blood count, 304
brain scan and EEG, 304
skull X-rays, 304
spinal tap, 304–305
Health care: choosing a hospital,
7–14
control of, 391–392
correction of social ills and, 393–
395
cost of, 391, 393–395
federally enforced guidelines,
391–392
future trends, 387–397
moral commitment to, 390
peer review, 45–47, 394
physician-patient relationships,
73–78, 395–397
right to, 388–392
Health foods, 206–207

Health Maintenance Organizations (HMO's), 45–46
Hearing loss, 279–282
  conductive and sensorineural, 280–281
  hearing aids, 281
  surgical treatment, 281
Heart attacks, 115, 119–132
  cardiopulmonary resuscitation, 89
  cause of collapse, 89
  monitoring, 126–127
  myocardial infarction, 120
  pacing and pacemakers, 127
  sickle-cell abnormalities and, 343
  (*See also* Coronary artery disease)
Heart disease, 115–140
  angina, 120–121
  arrhythmias, 124, 126
  atherosclerosis, 116, 119–121
  chest pains, 117–119
    angina, 120–121
  children and infants, 116
  choosing a doctor, 116–117
  congenital, 116
  coronary artery disease, 116, 119–132
    (*See also* Coronary artery disease)
  coronary care units, 126–127
  digitalis, 136
  diuretics, 136–137
  electrical conduction system, 115–116, 135
    abnormalities, 138
    temporary pacing, 127
  electrocardiograms, 69, 122
  extra or early beats, 138
  functional parts of heart, 115
  heart attacks (*see* Heart attacks)
  heart failure (congestive heart failure), 124, 134–137
  heart murmurs, 116, 139–140
  ischemia, 120, 170
  monitoring heart attacks, 126–127
  myocardial infarction, 120
  pain, 120–121, 170, 335
  palpitations, 137–139
  paroxysmal atrial tachycardia, 138

pericardium, 116
  preventive approach, 129
  "pump failure," 127–128
  rapid heart rates, 137–138
  rheumatic heart disease, 132–134, 356
  rhythm disorders, 124, 126
  risk factors, 129–132
    diabetes, 130
    exercise and obesity, 131
    heredity, 129–130
    increased cholesterol and triglycerides, 130–131
  surgery, 34
    coronary bypass, 124–125
  treatment, 126–128
    counterpulsation (mechanical assists), 127–128
Heart failure (congestive heart failure), 124, 134–137
  symptoms, 135–136
  therapy, 136–137
    diuretics, 136–137
Heart murmurs, 139–140
Heart specialists, 116–117
  cardiologists, 117
Heartburn, 121, 170
  reflux esophagitis, 170–172
Heat exhaustion or prostration, 113
Heimlich, Dr. Henry, 91
  maneuver in choking problems, 91
Hematologists, 27, 247
Hematology, 27
Hematuria (blood in urine), 376–378
Hemoglobinopathy, 343
Hemophilia, 299
Hemorrhoids, 35, 165, 185, 305–306
  surgical removal, 306
Heparin (anticoagulant drug), 366
Hepatitis, 175–179
  alcoholic, 178–179
  blood transfusions and, 176
  prevention of, 176
  treatment with gamma globulin, 176
  viral or "infectious," 175–176
Hepatologists, 175

Hereditary diseases (*see* Genetic counseling)
Hiatus hernia, 170–172
High blood pressure (*see* Hypertension)
Hip replacement surgery, 248–250
Hives, 244
HMO's (Health Maintenance Organizations), 45–46
Hospitals, 7–14
  accreditation, 8
  anesthesiology department, 56
  cancer expertise, 156–157
  choosing, 7–14
  coronary care units, 126–127
  emergency rooms, 36–37, 70, 328
  evaluating, 11–12
  federal health plans, 394
  interns and residents, 9, 36
  medical staff, 7–14
  nonprofit community vs. proprietary, 10–11
  patient care, 9–10
  selection of, 7–14
    geographical convenience, 10
  sources of information about, 12–14
  surgical environment, 56–57
  teaching, 8–10, 29
    affiliation with medical schools, 8–9
Human menopausal gonadotropin (HMG–Pergonal), 319
Hyperactive children, 306–308
  diagnosis, 306–307
  treatment with stimulant drugs, 307–308
Hypercapnia, 143
Hyperlipidemias, 130–131
Hypersensitivity reactions: liver disease, 176–177
  skin problems, 350
Hypertension (high blood pressure), 308–312
  atherosclerosis and, 310–311
  diagnosis, 309–310
    systolic/diastolic pressure, 309–310
  "essential hypertension," 311
  eye problems and, 310–311

  headaches and, 304
  heart disease and, 130, 135, 310–311
  hemorrhagic strokes and, 310–311, 359
  kidney failure and, 310–311
  nosebleeds, 111
  obesity and, 323
  treatment, 311–312
    drug therapy, 312
    low-salt diet, 312
Hypnosis, 325, 355
Hypoglycemia, 312–315
  diagnosis, 313
    glucose tolerance test, 313
  low blood sugar, 312–315
  treatment, 313–314
Hypoxemia, 143
Hysterectomies, 215
  vaginal and abdominal, 215, 219

Ileal bypass surgery, 325
Immunizations, 315–317
  keeping records of, 317
  measles, 316
  polio, 316
  recommended schedule for children, 315
  rubella, 316–317
  smallpox, 316
  tetanus, 317
  tuberculosis, 217
Immunology, 152–153
Impedance studies, 365
Impetigo (skin infection), 374
Independent Practitioners under Medicare: Report to Congress, 38
Infectious diseases, 27–28, 187–194
  "common cold," 190–191
  distinguishing bacterial from viral, 187–191
  "flu shots," 190–193
  laboratory tests, 188–189
  local infections, 191–192
  patient's history, 188
  symptoms, 189
  treatment, 189–190
  upper respiratory infections, 190–191

use of unnecessary antibiotics,
  187–189
use of vitamin C, 192, 205–206
Infertility, 317–320
  artificial insemination, 319–320
  clomiphene (Clomid) for, 266, 319
  definition of, 317–318
  diagnosis and treatment, 318–319
  incidence of, 317–318
Inflammatory bowel disease, 172–
  174
Informed consent, for surgical procedures, 56–57
Inhalation therapists, 13
Insect bites, allergic reactions, 242–
  243
Insomnia, 285
Insulin, 275–276
Internal medicine, 26–29
  cardiology, 26, 134
  endocrinology, 26–27
  gastroenterology, 27
  hematology, 27
  infectious disease, 27–28
  nephrology, 28
  neurology, 29
  oncology, 28
  pulmonary disease, 28
  rheumatology, 28–29
Internists, 26–29, 41
  fees, 61
  "fellowship" training, 26
Interns and residents, 6, 9, 22
  compensation, 60
  emergency room staffs, 36–37
Intestines
  cancer, 162
  inflammatory bowel disease, 172–
    174
  regional enteritis, 173
  ulcerative colitis, 173
  (*See also* Gastrointestinal diseases)
Ischemic heart disease, 120, 170
Itching (pruritus), 353
IUD's (intrauterine devices), 267–
  268

Jewish people, Tay-Sachs disease
  and, 297–298
Joint diseases, 28

arthritis, 247–251
  surgery, 248–250
    knee replacements, 250
    "total hip replacement," 248–
      250
Joint injuries, 104–106
  emergency treatment, 104–106
  knee joint, 105
  management controversies, 106
  severe, 105–106
  sprains, 104–106
  waiting period, 104–105
  x-ray studies, 105

Kaiser-Permanente plan, 45
Kidney diseases, 28, 35
  cancer, 152
  diabetes and, 278–279
  glomerulonephritis, 374–375
  hypertension and, 311
  strep infections and, 132, 356
  tumors, 378
Kidney stone formation, 206, 377–
  378
Kimmelstiel-Wilson disease, 229
Knee injuries, 105
  replacement surgery, 250

Laboratory tests, 36
  complete blood count, 188
  infectious diseases, 188–189
  urinalysis, 188
Lacerations (cuts), 106–110
  emergency treatment, 106–110
  grafting tissue, 107
  healing factors, 107–108
  suturing, 106–108
  tetanus booster shots, 108–110
  wound care, 107–108
Lahey Clinic (Boston), 45
La Leche League, 334
Laparoscopy technique, 219–220
L-dopa for Parkinson's disease,
  337–338
Lecithin, 208
Legal concerns and medical decisions, 75–76
  informed consent, 56–57
Leukemia, 27
  drug therapy, 155

Lithium, 288
Liver disease, 175–179
　alcoholic, 178–179
　avoidance of birth control pills,
　　265
　cancer, 179
　cirrhosis, 177–178
　hepatitis, 175–177
　hypersensitivity reactions, 176–177
"Low blood sugar," 312–315
　(See also Hypoglycemia)
Lung disease, 28, 141–150
　cancer, 147–148, 152
　chronic obstructive (bronchitis
　　and emphysema), 28, 143–
　　146
　　causes, 143–144
　　effect of air pollution, 145
　　effects of smoking, 142–145, 354
　　prevention, 144–146
　　pulmonary function tests, 145
　　symptoms, 143
　　treatment, 144–145
　effect of smoking, 142–145, 147–
　　148, 154–155, 354
　pneumonia, 146–147
　symptoms, 142–143
　tuberculosis, 148–150
Lungs, 141–142
　blood clots, 94, 118, 142
　breathing and respiration, 142
　chest pains, 118
　effect of heart failure, 135–136
　exchange of gases, 141–142
　fluid in, 142
　functional components, 141–142
　infections, 187
　pulmonary edema, 136, 142
　pulmonary embolus, 367–368
　thoracic surgery, 34

Malpractice suits, 76
Mann, Dr. George, 320–322
Mammography, 225
Mastoid infections, 283
Mayo clinic, 45, 169
Measles, vaccine for, 316
Medic-Alert identification, 243
Medical practice, changing pat-
　terns, 43–46

group practice, 43–46
Medical problems, 79–82
　clinical information, 80, 82
　confusion of opinions, 79–80
　"double blind" studies, 80
　"good evidence," 80
　sources of information for con-
　　sumers, 82, 399–401
Medical schools and teaching
　hospitals, 8–10
Medical societies, 17
　grievance committees, 65
Medical specialists (see Specialists,
　medical)
Medicare and Medicaid, 293
Meningitis, 305
Menopause: bleeding problems,
　216, 234, 238
　hormone-deficient status, 236
Mental disorders (see Emotional
　illness)
Mental health clinics, 286–287
Mental health professionals, 33,
　286–287
Metabolism rate, 198
　abnormal, 28, 296
　BMR (basal metabolism rate),
　　370
Migraine headaches, 303–304
Milk, nutritional value, 201, 207–
　208
Mongolism (Down's syndrome), 296,
　299, 333
Mouth: bleeding from, 184–185
　cancer, 152
　mouth-to-mouth breathing, 87
Multiple sclerosis, 29
Muscle strain and low-back pain,
　252–253
Myelograms, 255
Myocardial infarction, 120
Myringotomies, 283

National Academy of Sciences, Food
　and Nutrition Board, 198
National Cancer Institute, 157, 228
National Genetics Foundation, 287
National health care program, 387–
　396
　control of, 391

cost, 393–395
    social needs and, 394–396
National Institutes of Health, 157,
    362
National Research Council, 198
Near-drowning, emergency care, 94
Neck problems, radial neck surgery,
    32
Nephrologists, 28, 373
Nephrology (kidney disease), 28
Nerves, disorders, 29
    repair of, 35
    plastic surgery, 54
Neurological examinations, 361
Neurologists, 29, 305, 361
Neurology, 29
Neuromas, acoustic, 281
Neuropathies, 278
Neurosurgeons, 29, 99, 256–258,
    305, 361
    disk surgery, 32
New England Journal of Medicine,
    265, 288, 320
Nixon, Richard M., 60
Noise pollution, 282
Nosebleeds (epistaxis), 110–111
    emergency treatment, 110–111
Nurses, 40
    educational programs for, 11
    source of information about
        hospitals, 13
    visiting, 71
Nutrition, 194–209
    balanced diets, 198–200
    calories, 196–198
    carbohydrates, 200–201
    fats, 203–204
    health foods, 206–207
    other nutrients, 207–209
    proteins, 201–202
    safe and effective, 209
    vitamins, 204–206
    (*See also* Diet and nutrition)

Obesity, 320–326
    body metabolism and, 321
    changing basic eating habits, 322,
        326
    in childhood, 322
    diabetes and, 324

heart disease and, 131–132, 323
    hypertension and, 323
    influence on health, 320–326
    pregnancy and, 323–324
    treatment, 320, 324–326
        appetite suppressant drugs,
            324–325
        behavior modification, 324
        diets, 325
        exercise, 325–326
        group therapy, 324, 326
        hypnosis, 325
        ileal bypass surgery, 325
Obstetrical care, 326–335
    amniocentesis, 333
    birth control pills, 332–333
    breast feeding, 334–335
    emergencies and complications of
        delivery, 328
    family-centered maternal care,
        327–328
    fetal monitoring and care, 333–
        334
    first three months, 332–333
    high-risk pregnancies, 329–331
    home vs. hospital deliveries, 327
    nutrition and weight gain, 323–
        324, 331–332
    prenatal care, 329–331
    prepared (natural childbirth),
        328–329
    risk of abnormalities in, 332–333
    (*See also* Pregnancy)
Obstetricians, 29–30
Obstetricians-gynecologists, 212–213
Obstetrics, 30
Oncologists, 156
Operating-room technicians, 13
Ophthalmologists, 30–31, 289, 391
    training and expertise, 31
Ophthalmoscope, 28
Opticians, 31
Optometrists, 30
Oral contraceptives (*see* Birth-
    control pills)
Oral surgeons, 23
Organic foods, 207
Orthodontists, 23
Orthopedic surgeons, 31–32, 256–
    258

Orthopedic surgeons (*cont.*)
  joint injuries, 104, 106
Orthopedists, 31–32
Osteoarthritis, 253
Osteomalacia, 208
Osteopaths, 37–38
Osteoporosis, 237
Otolaryngologists, 280
Otoscopy, 282

Pacing and pacemakers, 127
Pain, 335–336
  "intractable pain," 336
  investigation of cause, 335–336
  (*See also* Back pain)
Palpitations, 137–139
  extra or early beats, 138
  paroxysmal atrial tachycardia,
    138–139
  sinus tachycardia, 137
  therapy, 139
Pancreas, cancer of, 162
Pap smears, 30, 68, 213–214, 234–
    236
  screening method, 233
Paramedical personnel, 40
Parkinson's disease, 29, 337–338
  L-dopa for, 337–338
Paroxysmal atrial tachycardia, 138–
    139
Pathologists, 13, 36, 63
Patients (*see* Physician-patient re-
    lationships)
Pediatricians, 32, 116, 156
  genetic counseling by, 297
  primary care functions, 41
Pediatrics, subspecialties, 32
Pedodontists, 23–24
Peer review, 45–47, 394
Pelvic area: examinations, 30, 213–
    214
  Pap smears, 30, 68, 213–214, 234–
    236
  pelvic inflammatory disease
    (P.I.D.), 381
Penicillin, 77–78
  for bacterial pneumonia, 147
  for strep throat, 133–134, 365–357
  for venereal disease, 383–384

(*See also* Antibiotics)
Pergonal (infertility drug), 319
Periodontists, 24, 272
Phenylbutazone, 180
Phlebitis, 362, 368
  (*See also* Thrombophlebitis)
Phlebograms, 365
Physiatrists, 362
  physical therapy and rehabilita-
    tion, 36
Physical examinations, 67–69
  annual, 67–69
  blood pressure checks, 68
  blood sugar tests, 69
  breast exam, 68
  chest X-rays, 69
  cholesterol and triglyceride tests,
    69
  ECG (heart tracings), 69
  glaucoma testing, 68
  Pap smears, 68
  rectal, 162, 339–340
  skin tests for TB, 150
Physical therapists, 13, 36, 362
Physician assistants, 40
Physician-patient relationships, 73–
    78
  actual encounter (first visit), 78
  art of medicine, 75–78
    interpreting evidence, 74
  medical decisions, 74–78
    legal concerns, 75–76
    malpractice suits, 76
    patient anxiety and, 77–78
    social status and, 76–77
Physicians:
  emergency-room, 36–37, 389
  evaluating doctors, 8, 11–12, 15–
    19
    checking on competency, 16–19
    continuing education, 17–19
    hospital affiliations, 7, 17, 48
    published papers, 17
    sources of information about,
      17
    teaching appointments, 17
    training and boards, 15–17, 26
  family physician movement, 18,
    25–26, 40–41, 81

fees (*see* Fees and fee schedules)
hospital-based, 7–14
house calls, 70–71
interns and residents, 9, 36
licensing requirements, 15–18
recertification, 18
listed by specialty, 21–38
national health care program,
380–392
peer review, 45–47, 394
selection of, 47–49
(*See also* Choosing a doctor)
specialists, 21–38
"Pill, The," 262–267
(*See also* Birth control pills)
Pink eye, 291
Planned Parenthood, 269, 318
Plastic surgeons and surgery, 35,
54–55, 259
cosmetic surgery, 55–56
fees, 55, 64
"plastic techniques," 54–55
radial neck surgery, 32
skin tumors, 352
Pleurisy, 118, 142
Pneumoencephalograms, 304
Pneumonia, 28, 118, 146–147, 187,
190
"atypical," 147
early diagnosis, 146
treatment with penicillin, 147
Poison Information Center, 100–101
Poisons and poisoning, 100–101,
375
emergency treatment, 100–101
Polio vaccinations, 316
Polyps, in colon, 165
Practice of medicine, 43–46
changing patterns, 43–46
group practice, 43–46
individual practice, 43
partnership arrangements, 44
referral practice, 43
Pregnancy, 326–335
breast feeding, 334–335
detecting problems, 298–300
family-centered maternity care,
327–328

fetal monitoring and care, 333–
334
first three months, 332–333
danger from medications, 332–
333
genetic counseling, 296–298
German measles (rubella), 300–
302
high-risk pregnancy, 330–331
home vs. hospital deliveries, 327
hormonal tests, 265
nutrition and weight gain, 198,
324, 331–332
obesity and, 323–324
prenatal care, 329–331
prepared (natural) childbirth,
328–329
role of amniocentesis, 239, 288–
289, 333
(*See also* Obstetrical care)
Preventive medicine, 45–46
Primary care, 39–41, 80–81
"crisis," 39–41
definition, 81
family physicians, 39
"good primary care physician,"
80–81
paramedical personnel, 40
Primary care physicians, 21, 49,
323
allergy problems, 245
fees, 63
recommendations for surgery, 53–
54
role of internists or pediatricians,
39–41
for women's health problems,
212–213
Proctologists, 35, 306
Progesterone, 238, 266
Propanalol, for migraine headaches, 303
Prostate disease, 338–340
cancer, 152, 340
prostate gland, 338
prostatism, 339
prostatitis (infection), 338–339
surgery, 35, 340
tumors, 339–340

Prostate disease (*cont.*)
BPH (benign prostatic hypertrophy), 339–340
Proteins in diet, 201–202
Pruritus (itching), 353
Psoriasis, severe, 349
Psychiatrists, 15, 33, 286
Psychologists, 33, 286
Psychotherapy, 288–289
Pulmonary disease (lung disease), 28
Pulmonary edema, 136
Pulmonary embolus (blood clot to lungs), 94, 367–368
Pulse, method of taking, 86
Pyelograms, 372–373
intravenous (I.V.P.), 372
retrograde, 372–373

Radiation therapy, 155
Radiologists, 13, 36, 63
Rashes, skin, 352–353
Rectocele, 218
Rectum: bleeding from, 165, 184–185
cancer of, 162, 164–166, 339
early diagnosis important, 185
examinations, 339–340
for appendicitis, 163
cancer of colon and rectum, 164
tumors of, 35, 339
Reflux esophagitis (heartburn), 170–172
Regional enteritis, 173
therapy, 36, 362
Rehabilitation and physical therapy, 36, 362
Reproductive system, 29–30
(*See also* Women's health problems)
Respiratory technicians, 13
Respiratory tract infections, 28
strep infections, 132–133, 356
upper, 132, 190–191
Rheumatic heart disease (rheumatic fever), 132–134, 374
acute phase of (rheumatic fever), 133
cause of heart failure, 135

chronic phase, 133
prevention of, 132–134
strep infections and, 132–133, 356–357
treatment, 133–134
penicillin and salicylates, 133–134
Rheumatoid arthritis, 28–29, 247–248
gold therapy, 248
Rheumatologists, 28, 248
Rheumatology (diseases of the joints), 28–29
Rhinitis, allergic, 244
Rhythm method of birth control, 269
Rib injuries, emergency treatment, 112–113
Rickets, 208
Risk factors in heart disease, 129–132
Root canal treatments, 22–23
Rubella (German Measles), 300–302
blood tests, 300–301
problem of exposure in pregnant women, 201–203, 317
vaccine, 300–302, 316–317

Salicylates, 133–134, 366
Salt intake, 208, 312
Scan studies, 304, 365, 368
Scopolomine, 328–329
Schweitzer, Albert, 396–397
Seizure disorders, 340–342
in children, 342
treatment, 95, 341
Shock:
definition, 357
emergency treatment, 95–96, 288
sickle-cell abnormalities, 343
(*See also* Strokes)
Sickle-cell abnormalities, 343–346
causes, 343–44
diagnosis and treatment, 345–346
screening tests, 344–345
sickle-cell anemia, 343
sickle-cell trait, 297, 343–344
Sigmoidoscopic examination, 161, 306
Silicosis, 144, 149

Sinus infections, 346–347
  sinusitis, 346–347
Sinus tachycardia, 137–138
Skin grafts, 35
  after burns, 103–104
Skin problems, 347–353
  baldness (alopecia), 258–259
  boils and carbuncles, 350–351
  cancer, 152, 154, 351–352
  dermatologists, 24–25, 259, 348
  diabetes and, 278–279
  eczematous dermatitis, 350
  itching (pruritus), 353
  manifestations of underlying
    disease, 350
  "moles," 352
  rashes, 244, 352–353
    allergy problems, 244
  severe acne, 349
  severe psoriasis, 349
  tumors, 351–352
  "moles," 352
Skin tests: for allergic reactions,
    244
  for tuberculosis, 150
Sleeping medications, 288
Smallpox vaccinations, 316
Smoking, 180, 323, 353–355
  heart disease and, 130, 354
  lung cancer and, 142–143, 147–
    148, 354
  medical reasons for stopping,
    353–355
  hypnosis for, 355
  weight gains and, 323, 355
Sore throats, 355–357
  (See also Strep infections)
Specialists, medical, 21–38, 305
  allergists, 21–22
  anesthesiologists, 36
  dentists, 22–24
  dermatologists, 24–25
  emergency-room physicians, 36–
    37
  general practitioners, 25–26
  GI diseases, 159–160, 172
  heart disease, 116–117, 139
  hospital-based, 35–37
  internists, 26–29
  neurologists-neurosurgeons, 29

obstetricians-gynecologists, 29–30
oncologists, 156
ophthalmologists, 30–31
orthopedists (orthopedic sur-
    geons), 31–32
osteopaths, 37–38
otolaryngologists (ENT specialists),
    32
pathologists, 36
pediatricians, 32
psychiatrists, 33
surgeons, 33–35
training and boards, 16–18
Spinal cord disorders, 29
  disk disease, 254–257
Spinal taps, 304–305
Spondylolysis or spondylolisthesis,
    254
"Sprain" injuries, 104–106
Sterilization procedures, 261–262
Steroids, 180
Stomach: cancer, 152, 162
  hiatus hernia, 170–172
  reflux esophagitis, 170–172
Strep infections, 356–357
  aggressive treatment of, 356–357,
    374
  diagnosis and treatment, 356–357
  kidney disease and, 132, 374
  rheumatic fever and, 132–134
  streptococcal bacteria, 356–357
  throat cultures, 356
  treatment, 134, 356–357, 374
  upper respiratory tract, 132, 356
  virus causes, 357
Strokes (cardiovascular accidents),
    357–362
  anticoagulant drugs and surgery,
    360–361
  causes, 358–359
  cerebral angiography, 361
  cerebral embolus, 358
  definition, 357–358
  emergency treatment, 94
  hemorrhages, 359
  hypertension and, 311
  "location" of symptoms, 359
  neurological symptoms, 357–358
  prevention, 359–361
  rehabilitation, 362

Strokes *(cont.)*
 sickle-cell abnormalities and, 343
 thrombosis, 358
 transient ischemic attacks, 359–
  361
 treatment, 94, 360–362
Surgery and surgeons, 15, 33–35
 abdominal, 219–220
 anesthesia administration, 56
 arthritis, 248–250
 board-certified, 52–53
 cancer, 155–156
 cardiac, 34, 57, 125, 133–134
  coronary artery bypass, 124–126
 colostomies, 166
 competency of surgeons, 52–54
 disk disease, 32, 256–257
 ear, nose and throat, 23, 32
 female problems, 214–220
  cystocele, 217
  D & C (dilation and curettage),
   215–216
  endometriosis, 217
  fibroids, 216–217
  laparoscopy technique, 219–
   220
  malpositioned uterus, 218
  procedures to restore pelvic
   anatomy, 217–218
  sterilization procedures, 220
  urinary stress incontinence,
   219–220
  uterine prolapse, 218
 gall bladder, 169
 general surgeons, 33–34
 high-risk, 57–58
 hospital environment, 56–57
 hysterectomies, 215, 219
 ileal bypass, 325
 "informed consent" requirements, 56–57
 minor, 53
 necessary and non-necessary, 51–
  52
  risks versus benefits, 57
  second opinion advisable, 51–52
 neurosurgery, 29, 361
 oral, 23
 orthopedic, 31–32, 256–258

 plastic, 23, 35, 54–56
 proctologists, 35
 prostate tumors, 35, 340
 radial neck, 32
 recertification requirements, 18
 referrals by primary care physicians, 53–54
 surgical environment and, 56–57
 thoracic, 34
 urologists, 28, 35
 vascular, 34–35, 361
**Syncope (fainting), emergency
 treatment, 95**
Syphilis, 380, 382–384
 diagnosis and treatment, 383–384
  blood tests, 383–384
 stages of the disease, 382–383
Syrup of ipecac, 100–101

Tay-Sachs disease, 296, 297, 299
Teaching hospitals, 8–10, 29
 affiliation with medical school,
  8–9
Teeth, care of, 270–272
Tendon repair, 35, 54
Tests and testing
 "double blind," 80
 legal concerns, 75–76
 unnecessary, 78
 (See also under name of disorder)
Tetanus immunization, 108–110
 children, 109
 vaccine, 317
Thermography, 226
Thoracic surgeons, 34
Throat, sore, 355–357
 cultures, 356
 (See also Strep infections)
Thrombolytic drugs, 366
Thrombophlebitis, 362–368
 cause and prevention, 364
 chronic venous insufficiency, 368
 of deep veins, 363–368
 distinction between bruise and,
  362–363
 pulmonary embolus, 367–368
 of superficial veins, 363
 symptoms, 365
 terminology, 362

treatment, 365–367
anticoagulant drugs, 366
surgical intervention, 367
thrombolytic drugs, 366
Thrombosis, 358
cerebral, 358
coronary, 358
Thrombus, 362
Thyroid disease, 27, 370–372
cancer of thyroid gland, 371
diagnosis and treatment, 370–372
effect on metabolism, 370
overactive (hyperthyroid), 138,
370
underactive (hypothyroid), 370–
371
Tissue specimens, interpreting, 36
Tolbutamide, 276–277
Tonsillectomy and adenoidectomy,
369–370
indications for surgery, 369–370
TOPS (Take Off Pounds Sensibly),
324
Toxins, hypersensitivity reaction,
177
Tracheitis, 141
Tranquilizers, 308
for emotional illness, 287–289
hypersensitivity reactions, 177
major and minor, 287–288
Transient ischemic attacks (TIA's),
359–361
Triglycerides and heart disease, 69,
130–131
Tubal ligation, 261
Tuberculosis, 148–150
chest X-rays, 148–150
prophylactic drug therapy, 149–
150
skin tests, 149–150, 317
symptoms, 148–149
Tuberculosis vaccine (BGG), 153
Tumors, 152
benign, 152
fibroid, 216–217
hospital tumor committees, 156
review of cases, 156–157
tumor registry, 157
malignant, 152

prostate, 339–340
rectal, 339
skin, 351–352
urinary tract, 378

UGDP (University Group Diabetes
Program), 276
Ulcers, 179–182
causes, 180
symptoms, 180
treatment, 180–181
antacids, 181
avoidance of irritants, 180–181
diet, 181
surgery, 181–182
Ultrasound studies, 365
Unconscious patients, moving, 97
Urinalysis, 372
Urinary tract problems, 28, 372–378
"bladder" infections, 376–377
cancer, 152
choice of doctor, 373
glomerulonephritis, 374–375
hematuria (blood in urine), 376–
378
identification of bacteria involved, 375–376
kidney stones, 377–378
surgery, 35
symptoms, 375
tests and testing, 372–373
cystoscopy, 373
intravenous pyelograms, 372
retrograde pyelograms, 372–373
treatment, 375–377
tumors, 378
urinary tract infections, 375–377
Urologists, 28, 35, 61–62, 373
for infertility problems, 318
Urticaria, 244
Uterus:
cancer of, 152, 231–234
cause and risk, 232
screening and diagnosis, 232–
234
Pap smears, 233, 234–236
treatment, 235–236
fibroid tumors, 216–217
malpositioned ("tipped"), 218

Uterus *(cont.)*
uterine prolapse, 218

Vaginal discharge, 220
Varicose veins, 378–379
surgery, 379
Vascular surgeons, 34–35
Vasectomies, 35, 261–262
Venereal disease, 380–385
antibiotics for treatment, 382–383
clinic services, 383
gonorrhea (clap), 380–382
prevention of, 380–381
risk of, 380–382
screening tests, 384
syphilis, 380, 382–384
Venograms, 365
Vinyl chloride, 154
Viral infections, 187–191
allergic reactions, 244
gastroenteritis, 162
Vitamins, 198, 204–206
fat-soluble (A, D, E, and K), 204–205
fluoridated, 271
water-soluble (B.C.), 205
vitamin B-12, 206
vitamin C, 192, 205–206
vitamin E, 206
Vomiting: following head injury, 97–98
induced by syrup of ipecac, 100–101

Wax in ears, 283–284
Weight Watchers, 324
White, Dr. Paul Dudley, 129, 199
Womanly Art of Breastfeeding, The, 334
Women doctors for women, 213
Women's health problems, 211–239
breast cancer, 221–231
biopsies, 227–228
diagnosis and treatment, 226–230
monthly self-examinations, 223–225

common complaints, 220–221
cervicitis, 220
dyspareunia, 221
vaginal discharge, 220
menopause, 236–239
bleeding problems, 216, 238
estrogen replacement therapy, 237–238
hormone-deficient status, 236
postmenopausal bleeding, 234
pelvic exam, 213–214
role of obstetrician-gynecologist, 212–213
surgical treatment, 214–220
bleeding problems, 215–216
cystocele, 217
endometriosis, 217
fibroids, 216–217
malpositioned uterus ("tipped"), 218
procedures to restore pelvic anatomy, 217–218
rectocele, 218
urinary stress incontinence, 219
uterine prolapse, 218
uterine and cervical cancer, 231–234
cause and risk, 232
Pap smear, 233–236
screening and diagnosis, 232–234
treatment, 235–236
Wound care, 107–180
tetanus immunization, 108–110

X-ray and laboratory technicians, 13
X-ray studies, 36
barium, 165, 166, 171
breast cancer, 154
chest, 69, 148–150
GI diseases, 161
joint injuries, 105
mammography, 225
myelograms, 255
skull, 98–99, 304
thrombophlebitis, 365, 368